FIRST INTERNATIONAL SYMPOSIUM
ON ARTIFICIAL LENSIMPLANTATION

Editor

A.Th.M. VAN BALEN

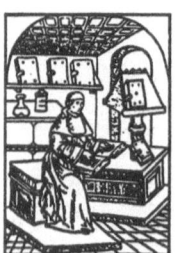

DR. W. JUNK B.V. PUBLISHERS, 1975
THE HAGUE   THE NETHERLANDS

DOCUMENTA OPHTHALMOLOGICA

PROCEEDINGS SERIES

VOL. VI

Editor

HAROLD E. HENKES

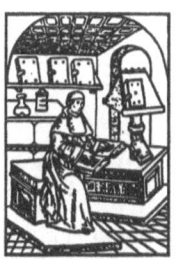

DR. W. JUNK B.V. PUBLISHERS, 1975
THE HAGUE   THE NETHERLANDS

ISBN-13: 978-90-6193-146-1   e-ISBN-13: 978-94-010-1952-1
DOI: 10.1007/ 978-94-010-1952-1

CONTENTS

PREFACE

In 1958, on the occasion of the centenary of the Koninklijk Nederlands Gasthuis voor Ooglijders at Utrecht, the Snellen medal was founded by the Board of the hospital in memory of PROF. DR. HERMAN SNELLEN SR. This medal should be presented each 5th year to a person of Dutch nationality, who had exceptionally distinguished himself in the field of ophthalmology.

The Snellen committee, of which I had the honour to be a member, was unanimous in their choice of the laureate of this award; it should be Dr. C.D. BINKHORST for his outstanding and ingenious work on the intra-ocular implant lens. BINKHORST, an exceptionally gifted eye-surgeon, started lens implantation in 1955, after he had studied Ridley's method in London. He introduced several improvements, and in 1957 developed his iris clip lens, in which fixation of the implant lens was provided by the iris diaphragm. The iris clip lens was followed in 1965 by the iridocapsular lens, intended for extracapsular extractions, while the iris clip lens was suitable for both intracapsular and extracapsular extraction. BINKHORST has earned a world reputation and ophthalmologists from all over the world come to the little towns of Terneuzen and Sluiskil in the province of Zeeland, to learn his technique.

Next came the idea to organize a special day for the presentation of the medal. The chairman of the committee, Dr. HOPPENBROUWERS, had a very busy job in organizing this clinical day, for which he invited several well-known authorities from abroad, and so this day grew out to the first international symposium on intraocular implant lenses in the world. More than 300 participants attended this meeting, and afterwards we thought that it might be beneficial to our colleagues to have the proceedings of this meeting appear in print.

Thanks are due to Miss LA BASTIDE, for typing out the panel discussion, and to Prof. HENKES and Dr. VAN BALEN, who took care of the editing and printing of the manuscript. We sincerely hope that this first symposium on intraocular implant lenses may provide usefull information on this still controversial subject.

PROF. DR. J.E. WINKELMAN,
Koninklijk Nederlands Gasthuis
voor Ooglijders,
Utrecht.

THE IMPLANTATION OF ARTIFICIAL LENSES IN TRAUMATIC CATARACT IN CHILDREN

A.TH.M. VAN BALEN

(Rotterdam)

ABSTRACT

The indication of iridocapsular lensimplantation in traumatic cataract in children is discussed. Some technical aspects of the operation and related complications are described. The results of 37 cases treated in the Rotterdam Eye Clinic are given.

The discussion about the implantation of acrylic lenses is still in full progress. I believe this is good and I hope that more critical studies will be done to evaluate the long term results. We are looking forward to the report of the Miami group. In the discussions however a clearcut discrimination has to be made between the intracameral lenses and the irissupported lenses because it has now been established clearly enough that the complications to be expected in the implantation of these two kind of lenses are different, to say the least.

Although the implantation of acrylic lenses in children seems to be premature, because evaluations of results over more than 15 years are scarce, in my opinion the implantation of a pseudophakos in traumatic cataract in children is an absolute indication. The risk of amblyopia, the difficulties of wearing contactlenses, the residual aniseikonia of 5 - 10% (OGLE & BURIAN, 1958), the vertical prismatic effects, the frequent loss of contactlenses are all causes of early abandoning of this correction and therefore of poor longtermresults (RIDLEY, 1953 and RUBINSTEIN, 1960).

All the difficulties are summarized by JANE JOHNSTON, in 1972. In the discussion on BINKHORST's paper in the 3rd European Congress I mentioned 15 cases of traumatic cataract resulting in good aphakic vision. Of these 15 children of over 5 years old six children could not wear contactlenses, nine children could wear the contactlens with success, six had binocular vision, two had convergent and one divergent strabismus. Two of the six children with good binocular vision did not wear the contactlens. The conclusion was: only four of fifteen cases of traumatic aphakia in children could be corrected with a contactlens. There are several reports of larger groups of unilateral aphakics corrected by contactlenses with rather poor results. These reports pertain all age groups and not only traumatic cataract. LEONARD & EVENS (1971) gave a very pessimistic report of only 5% succesfull corrections of unilateral cataract by contactlenses in a large group of young men. Perhaps the soft lenses will proof to be more

1

succesfull. In Rotterdam we do not have sufficient experience with this kind of contactlenses in children yet. DREIFUS (1970) however found only 10% binocular vision in children corrected with soft lenses.

The iridocapsular lens was designed by BINKHORST to use in extracapsular lensextraction and was meant to be inplanted in children and young adults. I will not describe the lens and the operationmethod because this has been done in extenso by BINKHORST and I stick to his operationtechnique quite strictly.

You all know that the platinum iridium loops have to be shifted in the cleft between the iris and the posterior capsule. Important points in view of the ultimate results are:

1. removal of lens material as soon as possible after the trauma or after the development of cataract and in the same operation implantation of the pseudophakos. When the perforation of the anterior lenscapsule by the trauma or by the discission has happened too long before the implantation you run the risk of the lensremnants becoming organized into strong fibrous material that cannot easily be removed.

2. removal of sufficient lensmaterial in order to avoid swelling of the lensremnants that would push forward a part of the pseudophakos.

3. removal of not too much lensmaterial in order to have sufficient fixation by iridocapsular adhesions.

In several cases of lensimplantation in traumatic cataract one can find white deposits on the pseudophakos during the first few weeks. They disappear spontaneously and we think that they consist of lensproteins.

When not sufficient adhesions between iris and posterior capsule of the lens have developed, one can find movements of the pseudophakos caused by the pupillary movements and atrophy of the pupillary border on the point where the lower loopattachment is resting on that border.

The iridocapsular lens apparently is too heavy for the support by the sphincter only. You can even have luxation of the pseudophakos usually after slight trauma. The movements of the pseudophakos can rubb off the pigment of the pigmentlayer of the iris. In three instances it can be necessary to do a secondary fixation of the iridocapsular lens to the iris by the transcorneal way.

Contra indications for iridocapsular lensimplantation are in my opinion:

1. rupture of the posterior capsule by the trauma or during the operation.

2. large iriscolobomata although in some instances it is possible to close the wound in the iris after implanting the lens in such a way that the lens is sufficiently supported. BINKHORST (1969) has given some examples of this procedure.

3. corneal scars that cause serious irregular astigmatism. It is difficult however to estimate the amount of astigmatism that will remain after the curing of the original corneal wound. I have seen a corneal scar of 10 diopters astigmatism and some irregularity one month after the suturing of the corneal wound flatten to a scar of two diopters astigmatism in the opposite direction without any irregularity 6 months afterwards.

The results of 37 implantations are shown in diagram I, of these 24 have a visual acuity of 0.5 or more. Interesting is that several cases of visual acuity less than o.5 still have binocular vision or even stereoscopic vision.

2

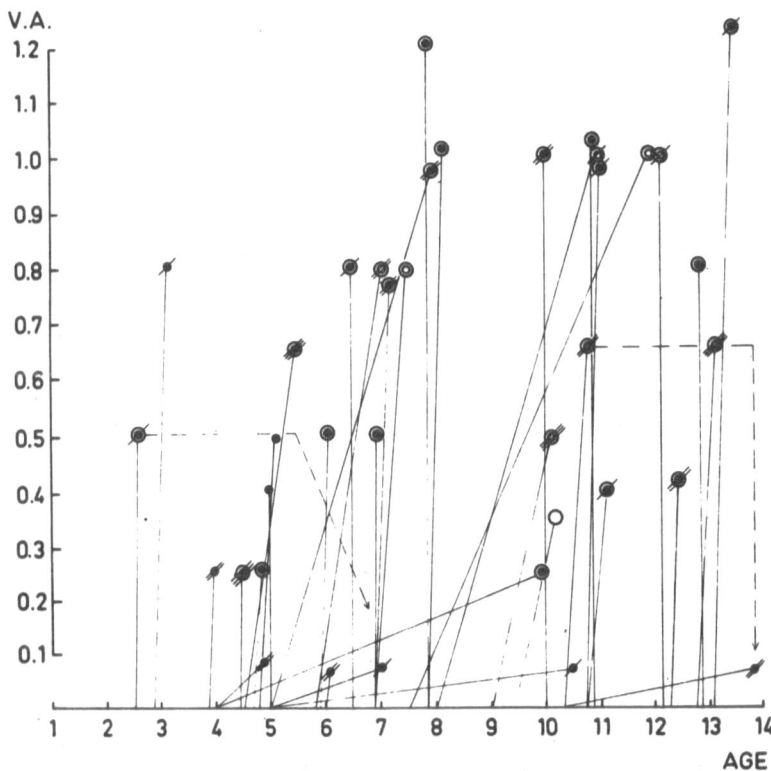

Diagram I

37 implantations

Visual acuity attained by lensimplantations in children with unilateral aphakia after operation for cataract caused by blunt O or perforating ● trauma.
Double contour ◎ means stereoscopic vision present. The inclination of the lines connecting the symbols with the abscis gives information about the interval between trauma and lensimplantation.

1 case in the diagram subsequently lost vision because of amblyopia due to an after cataract membrane (V.A. 0.5 → 0.1) and 1 case because of retinal detachment (V.A. 0.67 → 0.1). 2 cases are not included in the diagram; one because of insufficient control, one because of blunt trauma 6 days after implantation by which the pseudophakos was expressed from the eye through the ruptured operation wound. The results at this moment therefore are 39 implantations, 37 evaluated, 22 have V.A. of 0.5 or more.

As it is to be expected the visual acuity ultimately reached among other things depends on age and interval between trauma and implantation of the pseudophakos. The inclination of the lines connecting the symbols with the abscis in diagram I gives information about the duration of this interval.

Discission has to be done in quite a number of cases. In this group in about 60% and half of them more than once.

The discission of the posterior capsule and after cataract membrane is

3

not a difficult procedure when a pseudophakos is present. The discission needle is moved in between the iris and the border of the lens and the discission of the membrane is easier because it is more or less stretched by the loops of the pseudophakos and has less tendency than usual to move away from the point of your discission needle.

CONCLUSION

Although we still do not know whether the iridocapsular lens is tolerated longer than 10 years in the eye we strongly advise implantation of this lens in unilateral traumatic cataract in children because no other correction of unilateral aphakia in children gives good enough results as far as binocular vision is concerned.

REFERENCES

BINKHORST, C.D., GOBIN, M.H. & LEONARD, P.A.M. Posttraumatic artificial lens implants (pseudophakoi) in children. *Brit. J. Ophtal.* 53: *518* (1969).

BINKHORST, C.D., GOBIN, M.H. & LEONARD, P.A.M. Posttraumatic pseudophakia in children. *Ophthalmologica* 158: *284* (1969).

DREIFUS M. Clinical experience with hydrophilic contact lenses in children with unilateral aphakia. *Ophthalmologica* 161: *279* (1970).

JOHNSTON, J.B. Management of children in contact lenses. *Brit. Orthopt. J.* 29: *17* (1972).

LEONARD, P. & EVENS, L. La vision binoculaire dans l'aphakie unilaterale traumatique. *Bull. Soc. belge Ophtal.* 159: *697* (1971)

MILLS, P.V. & LEWIS, E.M.T. Scleral contact lens wear in unilateral aphakia. *Brit.J. ophthal.* 55: *116* (1971).

OGLE, K.N. BURIAN, H.M. & BANNON,R.E. On the correction of unilateral aphakia with contact lenses. *Arch. Ophthal.* 59: *639* (1958).

RIDLEY F. Contact lenses in unilateral aphakia. *Trans. Ophthal. Soc. U.K.* 73: *373* (1953).

RUBINSTEIN, K. Management of unilateral aphakia. *Brit. Orthopt. J.* 17: *82* (1960).

VANNAS, S. et al. Binocular vision in monocular aphakia correctible by contact lenses. *Acta Ophthal.* 50: *589* (1972).

Author's address:
A.Th.M. van Balen M.D.
Department of Ophthalmology
Erasmus University
Eye Hospital
Schiedamse Vest 180
Rotterdam.
The Netherlands

EXPERIENCES IN 100 ARTIFICIAL LENSIMPLANTATIONS AFTER INTRACAPSULAR LENSEXTRACTION

A.M. LEEMAN

(Amersfoort)

The fact that our honoured colleague Dr. C.D. BINKHORST received the Snellen-reward for his fundamental contribution in the field of intraocular implants, is not only a recognition of his own work, but it also is a milestone in the development of this special aspect of ophthalmology.

I feel honoured to have the opportunity to make a contribution on this special day.

The iriscliplens, promoted by BINKHORST, has not yet conquered the entire world and even in our own country the by JAFFE illustratively called 'incredibility gap' has not been bridged altogether. It nevertheless means something that in 1971 3024 intracapsular lensextractions done in the Netherlands on patients belonging to the obligatory insurance system, 381 were supplied with an iriscliplens (12 1/2%).

In the hospitals participating in the medical registration system (65%) even more implants were administered.

1971: 2702 intracapsular extractions of which 421 got implants, 15,6%.

1972: 3281 intracapsular extractions of which 548 got implants, 16,6%. In my opinion these figures illustrate that the possibilities of the iriscliplens is recognised by a number of able Dutch ophthalmologists. In 1971 of the 270 ophthalmologists working for the obligatory insurance system 168 were performing cataract extractions. Of these 168 surgeons 27 implanted 381 artificial lenses. It appears that the more implants are placed by these surgeons the less aphakic eyes they leave behind, showing their (over?) confidence in the method.

Members of the staff of the Royal Dutch Eye Hospital in Utrecht were rather critical of the possibilities of the method and made at first only use of implant surgery in some cases of traumatic cataract in children, knowing that without such therapy amblyopia has a good chance to develop.

When the results in those cases proved to be favourable I started in my private practice in Amersfoort to use implant lenses in selected cases of unilateral cataracts. In the beginning mostly after extracapsular lensextraction, later also after intracapsular lensextraction in the elderly patient, especially when it became possible to fixate the lenses in these cases so that the possibility of luxation of the implant diminished markedly. In the beginning I implanted only unilateral cases, but when these patients developed cataracts in the second eye and when the implantation of the first eye was

100% succesfull, I also implanted a pseudophakos in the fellow eye in a number of cases.

MATERIAL AND METHODS

In september 1973 I gathered 100 cases of implants after intracapsular lensextraction. These cases will be surveyed in this paper.
Number of cases in:
1969: 1
1970: 5
1971: 25
1972: 31
1973: 38. Three of the patients died during these 4 years. In two cases I refrained from implantation because of impeding vitreous-loss.

51 of the pseudophakoi were of the 4 loop type (BINKHORST). Of these 4 were kept in place by miotics only, 42 of them were vertically placed and fixated by connecting the two superior loops through an iridectomy by a nylon suture.

The remaining 5 were fixated by a perlon suture through the iris and 2 anterior loops of the lens.

The other 49 pseudophakoi were iriscliplenses modified by WORST, having only 2 horizontal posterior loops and at the 12 o'clock position an enlarged haptic part, containing 2 holes to be able to suture the lens to the iris.

Over 85% of the pseudophakic patients were over 70 years old. The remaining 15% were all unilateral cases and 20 bilateral implanted cases.

We compared the results with a group of 100 at random chosen healthy uncomplicated aphakic eyes.

SURGICAL PROCEDURE

Of course every possible measure should be taken to promote an optimal result. This means working with a well trained team, while the task of the assisting surgeon is almost as important as the main surgeon.

My associate, Dr. P.A.W. LINDENBURG, and I are always doing the surgery together, assisting each other during implant-surgery. Also of imminent importance is the availability of a skilled anaesthesist with special knowledge in the field of ophthalmic surgery, preferably using muscle relaxation.

In implant surgery one has to take special care to avoid dust and other particles, such as cotton, threads, to enter the eye. Of course all well known measures should be taken to promote the safety of the surgery such as the use of a Flieringa ring if indicated.

We use the normal ab externo procedure with a corneal based conjunctival flap and 10X0 nylon sutures to close the qound. To entrance safety in regard to implantation we came to do the iridectomy after implantation and not before lensextraction. When an iris suture is required we place this before the lensextraction.

When inserting the implant utmost care must be taken not to damage the

6

cornea endothelium nor the vitreal surface. One should never attempt lens-implantation in an eye with bulging vitreous.

When a preplaced iris suture is used it sometimes is difficult to avoid that the thread becomes tangled in one of the posterior loops of the pseudo-phakoi. When this happens it is difficult, but possible, to untangle the thread by cutting and reknotting it.

POSTOPERATIVE COMPLICATIONS

Shortly after the operation some difficulties can occur. Such as:
1. loss of anterior chamber
2. rise of intraocular pressure
3. luxation of the pseudophakos
4. corneal dystrophy
5. intra-ocular infection.

Sub.1. Loss of anterior chamber

The most frequent cause of loss of the anterior chamber in case of a lensimplant is aqueous block. This occurred in some cases especially when a two-loop cliplens of Worst was used. This complication was promoted by the use of miotics during operation and restoration of the anterior chamber by air.

In these cases the anterior chamber can readily be restored by the instillation of mydriatics. In only one instance shallowing of the anterior chamber was caused by leakage of the wound. Resuturing of the wound solved the problem. In this series we did not see one case of choroidal detachment. This was in contrast to 5 cases of choroidal detachment in the series of 100 aphakic eyes. I don't think this is due to a more meticulous closure of the wound in the implant cases. I am inclined to ascribe this to the prevention of a vitreous prolaps in the anterior chamber by the implant.

Sub.2. Rise of intraocular pressure.

This complication occurs nearly always in combination of loss of the anterior chamber by pupillary block. Restoration of the chamber solves the problem.

Apart from the first mentioned complication we found that in the first 5 to 7 postoperative days the intraocular pressure of the pseudophakic eye usually is somewhat elevated. I don't think this to be due to the use of steroids because as a rule the pressure normalises after a week, in spite of the continuation of steroids. Chymotrase is also out of the question as a cause because we don't use it routinely. Maybe it is due to the manipulation of the iris with disturbance of the pigmentlayer. To avoid damage to the eye we routinely give 500 mg diamox during the first week. The prolonged use of steroids in implant cases has brought us to a steroid test before surgery.

Sub.3. Luxation of the pseudophakos

Luxation of the pseudophakos the first postoperative days may happen. Readjustment by dilatation of the pupil is succesfull in most cases. When this proves impossible surgical intervention is mandatory but easy.

Sub.4. Corneal dystrophy

We have one case of corneal dystrophy developing directly after surgery. In this case the dystrophy was caused by an exfolation of the Descements membrane during surgery.

Sub.5. Intraocular infection

No case of intraocular infection did occur in our series. When this happens it perhaps may prove more difficult to cure than in cases without an intraocular foreign body.

LATE COMPLICATIONS

a. luxation of the pseudophakos
b. iritis
c. maculopathies) cystoid)senile
d. glaucoma
e. corneal dystrophy
f. retinal detachment.

Sub.a. Late luxation of the pseudophakos

This occurred in 11 eyes. Three of these were associated with a blow against the head.

Frequency	Type of fixation	Lens	Position	Number of eyes
1	miotics only	4 loops	horizontal	4
1	iris suture	4 loops	horizontal	5
2	loop connection	4 loops	vertical	42
7	iris suture	2 loops	horizontal	49

As can be seen the horizontal position and the iris suture are more associated with lens luxation as in the other cases. It should be stated here however that to prevent the occurrence of a high riding implant in the beginning I made the bite of the iris suture very small, which decreased the stability of frequency deminished. Nevertheless I am convinced that because of the predominant horizontal eye movements the luxation frequency of horizontally placed lenses will always tend to be higher than the vertical ones. Probably the new modification of Worst, with 2 vertically placed posterior loops and a haptic part at the 12 o'clock position, armed with a

8

blunt pin of platinum, that can be bent backwards, through an iridectomy inside of the posterior loop, will prove to be the best mode of fixation.

The more so because the nylon sutures proved to fragmentate after 3 to 4 years. This last type of lens combines an easy insertion in the eye with a reliable fixation. Dilatation of the pupil without promoting luxation of the lens is also possible.

Sub.b. Iritis

In one patient we saw 1 1/2 year after surgery an attack of acute iritis. Luckily this case could be cured in five weeks using dexamethasoon and scopolamine eyedrops. The visual acuity was also restored to normal (5/5). In 9 eyes we saw a prolonged low grade iritis. Four of the eyes became absolutely quiet 2 to 3 month after surgery. The other 4 eyes remained somewhat irritated. Three of them showed a deterioration of the visual acuity varying between 5/10 and 5/30, due to cystoid maculopathy.

Sub.c. Maculopathy

Cystoid maculopathy (Irvine Gass syndrome) is the most annoying complication associated with artificial lensimplantation. Unfortunately there seems to be no sign in the unoperated eye to predict this kind of complication. Most of the pseudophakic eyes with cystoid maculopathy show a low grade iritis the origin of which is unknown. In my opinion damage to the vitreal surface may prove to be of some importance in the onset of this phenomenon. As a rule eyes with cystoid maculopathy at the beginning show a deterioration of vision to approximately 0,25. In the course of 6 to 8 weeks most of these eyes recover a vision of 5/10 tot 5/5. Some of them, however, don't recover that much. In our series 4 eyes showed a diminished vision between 5/30 and 5/15, due to the Irvine Gass syndrome. This is slightly more than in the control group of aphakic eyes, where I found 3 of such cases. In the pseudophakic as well as in the aphakic group of eyes we saw 3 cases of senile dry maculopathy.

Sub.d. Elevation of the intraocular pressure

As said before we saw as a rule a moderate rise of intraocular pressure during the first postoperative week.

In 4 eyes, however, we found a prolonged elevation of pressure lasting more than 6 weeks and correlated with the use of steroids. Only one case showed a long lasting elevation of the pressure. This eye suffers also from a low grade iritis and cystoid maculopathy. Medication of 500 mg diamox kept the intraocular pressure within normal limits. Four cases of known glaucoma simplex needing pilocarpine 2% eyedrops 3 times daily, showed an elevated intraocular pressure after implant surgery. Two of these patients acquired microruptures in the sphincter pupillae during lensextraction preventing the pupil to obtain maximal miosis.

Sub.e. Corneal dystrophy

In our experience it is not uncommon to see some epithelial edema in the 2 postoperative weeks. Sometimes this edema persits for even a longer time. In most instances it is located near the limbus at the 12 o'clock position and it does not disturb the vision.

Apart from the already mentioned traumatic corneal dystrophy in this series uptil now we did not see any case of late corneal dystrophy.

Sub.f. Retinal detachment

This complication occurred in one eye. A sister of this patient also suffered from retinal detachment. Detachment surgery was in the first instance succesfull, but the detachment recurred after three months and proved irreparable because of the formation of starfolds.

OBTAINED RESULTS

The visual acuity of the implant cases, as compared to the aphakic cases, did not show much difference.

Visual acquity	Pseudophakia	Aphakia
5/4 − 5/6	86	84
6/10 − 5/10	6	8
5/5 − 5/20	3	3
5/30 − 5/50	3	2
1/10	2	3

BINOCULARITY

Of the 60 unilateral cases:

Four dots test		Flye test
54	positive	52
6	negative	8

Of the 20 bilateral cases:

Four dots test		Flye test
19	positive	18
1	negative	2

The choice which cases may benefit of implant surgery, depends on a carefull evaluation of the known and even unknown complications brought about by this kind of surgery.

In the first place implantation surgery entrances the risks for the eye during surgery, be it that in the hands of an experienced surgeon the extra risk is not very great.

Secondly we do not yet know for sure that in the long run no new complications may arise.

Thirdly it seems undeniable that the Irvine Gass syndrome presents itself somewhat more frequent in pseudophakic eyes. The other complications do not seem to be more frequent.

This leads to the conclusion that one should select his cases amongst the elderly patients especially those with unilateral cataracts. The fact that the elderly patient has the biggest problems to adapt him(her)self to the aphakic state, speaks for this agegroup. With growing experience maybe we come to handle less rigid criteria but I think for the time being it is a sound starting point. The younger the patient is, the stronger the indication (need of binocular view and other occupational requirement) should be.

Lensimplantation in the fellow eye of a pseudophakic eye should only be undertaken more than 6 months after the first implantation has been 100% succesfull and only in patients over 70 years of age.

Contraindications

1. all kinds of sick eyes
2. diabetes with angiopathy (legs and kidneys)
3. previous retinal detachment surgery
4. some congenital abnormalities.

Relative contraindications.

1. bilateral cataracts in infants and young adults
2. family history of retinal detachments
3. long standing diabetes without angiopathy
4. myopia of more than 6 diopters
5. shallow anterior chamber
6. rheumatoid arthritis, M. Bechterew etc.
7. corneal dystrophy.

Most of these listed contraindications speak for themselves. Some of them are quite arbitrary such as shallow anterior chamber. In these cases, after the lens has been removed, the depth of the anterior chamber as a rule becomes normal. In cases however with a suspect history, or even with prodromal symptomes of acute glaucoma, I would reject implant surgery.

When severe cornea guttata or even a clear case of Fuchs dystrophy has developed the decission becomes realy difficult. Cataract surgery alone in these cases may also provoke a deterioration of the dystrophy. In implant surgery the pseudophakos keeps the vitreous back, which may prevent a disastrous development. Also it must be kept in mind that corneal transplants have a better prognosis in pseudophakic eyes.

Of course when none of these contraindications is present the condition of the eye during surgery is of mandatory importance in the decision to proceed with an artificial lensimplantation or not. One should always tell the patient that one will take the final decision during surgery.

In conclusion I would say that, although artificial lensimplantation is correlated with a somewhat higher percentage of complications, in the hands of experienced surgeons it is a method which yields good results.

As long as contactlenses are not succesfull in all aphakics, lensimplantation is the method of choice in those cases were the optical advantages outweigh the risks.

One should not underestimate the optical handicaps of the aphakic eye so clearly described by ALLAN WOOD when judging the merits of implant surgery.

Author's address:
A.M. Leeman M.D.
Van Hogendorplaan 1
Amersfoort
The Netherlands

ULTRASONOGRAPHIC OCULOMETRY AND THE OPTICS OF THE EYE

H. GERNET

(Münster)

Abstracted and translated by A.TH.M. VAN BALEN

The Lecturer (G) expresses his gratitude for the invitation to speak about his work during the symposium in honour of Dr. C.D. BINKHORST.

Three years ago he met Dr. BINKHORST. Since then G. was able to observe not only his outstanding surgical technique but also his critical approach to the problem of aniseikonia. Both WORST and BINKHORST have stimulated G. in his work on the correction of aniseikonia.

Ultrasonographic oculometry has given ophthalmologists the opportunity to measure objectively and accurately the axial length of the eye and its relevant optical subdivisions, instead of estimating them on the theoretical basis of the schematic eye of Gullstrand.

Using ultrasonographic oculometry and appropriate formulas, one can calculate the dioptric value of the lens and the size of the retinal image. G and coworkers have given evidence that the dioptric value of the lens of the emmetropic eye is not 19.11 as in the Gullstrand eye, but 23,7 diopters.

G. congratulates Dr. BINKHORST with the fact that the dioptric value of 20.5 of this original implant lens, although empirically determined, largely corresponds with the calculated value for an emmetropic eye that is 1.5 diopter myopic after the implantation.

G. explains his method for calculating the specific strength of the implantation lens to suite a given eye.

G. discussed too a method for the correction of unilateral aphakia by the combination of an overcorrecting contact lens and a negative spectacle lens before the phakic eye.

He proposes this method as an alternative to lens implantation. He is sure that BINKHORST will welcome this addition to the therapeutical arsenal in the struggle to overcome the crippling effects of unilateral aphakia; an arsenal of which BINKHORST's outstanding contribution, now acknowledged and honoured by the Snellen award constitutes a major part.

Author's address:
H. Gernet
University Eye Clinic
Münster
B.R.D.

DISLOCATION AND ENDOTHELIAL CORNEAL DYSTROPHY (ECD) IN PATIENTS FITTED WITH BINKHORST LENS IMPLANTS (1958 - 1972)

M.E. NORDLOHNE

(Vlissingen)

Medio tutissimus ibis.
OVIDIUS.

Dislocation of the lens implant has been the pre-eminent complication in patients fitted with Ridley lens implants in the posterior chamber of the eye.

Endothelial corneal dystrophy (ECD) has been the pre-eminent complication in patients fitted with anterior chamber lens implants with angle fixation.

Binkhorst's iris clip lens and its modifications were designed to avoid both dislocation and ECD as far as possible and to get the best of both types of implants.

Dislocation and ECD will be discussed on the basis of the 694 iris clip lens implant operations carried out by BINKHORST up to 1-1-1972.

INCIDENCE OF DISLOCATION

Dislocation occurred in 53 eyes (7.64%) because of
1. inadequate loop length. The loop length may be defined as the largest dimension of the iris clip lens, that is the length of the line connecting the extremities of the diametrically opposed loops.

In the first 96 implants the anterior loop length was about 7 mm. In the next series of implants up to and including no. 180 (3-6-1965) it was about 8 mm. In the third series, up to and including no. 394, the anterior loop length was 9 to 9.5 mm (to prevent dislocation) and since then it has been maximally 8 mm (to prevent ECD).

The relationship between dislocation and loop length is shown in Fig. 1.

	loop length	number of eyes	number of eyes with dislocation	%
11-8-58 until 3- 8-62	approx. 7 mm	96	15	15.62
9-8-62 until 3- 6-65	approx. 8 mm	84	20	23.81
10-6-65 until 12-12-68	approx. 9 mm	214	5	2.34
9-1-69 until 31-12-71	8 mm	300	13	4.33
11-8-58 until 31-12-71		694	53	7.64

Fig. 1. Incidence of dislocation with respect to the loop length employed in 694 iris clip lens implant operations performed by BINKHORST.

It is a paradox that the percentage of dislocations in the first 8 mm series is larger than in the 7 mm series (23.81 against 15.62). However, it may be explained in part by the fact that 75.0% of the 7 mm series consisted of *secondary* implant operations where at a considerable period of time after the cataract extraction the behaviour of the pupil was known whilst 96.4% of the first 8 mm series consisted of *primary* implant operations where the behaviour of the pupil was a matter of speculation.

What is striking is that the high percentages of 15 and 23 and the low percentages of 2 and 4 are separated by the date of June 1965. This is the month in which routine installation of pilocarpine hydrochloride 2%, twice daily, was introduced as a post-operative routine. It coincided with the use of the longer loop length of 9 mm, too.

The difference between the two 8 mm series is mainly due to
a. routine instillation of pilocarpine hydrochloride 2%, twice daily, in the last group from the beginning, and
b. suturing of the superior loops to each other (46x) or suturing the loops to the iris (13x) in the second series.
2. insufficient miosis of the pupil, especially during darkness. Exact figures are not available.
3. blunt trauma. Three cases.

The incidence of dislocation with respect to the 1st, 2nd, 3rd, etc., hundred of implant operations, is shown in Fig. 2.

	implant operation date no. 100, 200, etc.	number of eyes	number of dislocations	
			total	first week only
1st hundred	20- 9-62	15	25	6
2nd hundred	7-10-65	20	24	3
3rd hundred	29-11-67	3	3	2
4th hundred	14- 2-69	2	5	–
5th hundred	26-11-69	6	6	5
6th hundred	15- 1-71	5	8	3
last 94	9-12-71	2	2	–
total 694		53	73	19

Fig. 2. Distribution of dislocations for every 100 cases amongst the 694 iris clip lens implant operations performed by BINKHORST.

The incidence of dislocation decreased considerably after June 1965 due to the pilocarpine medication, and as a result of the introduction of the loop length of *9.00* mm. However, it increased slightly after 1-1-1969 when the loop length was changed to *8.00* mm.

The consequences of dislocation were relatively slight. In 3 cases (0.43%) dislocation occurred twice, and together with its repositionings it may have contributed to the development of ECD; in 2 cases (0.29%) anterior dislocation of one loop caused local corneal oedema which disappeared after repositioning.

Cases with ECD may be divided into 3 groups:

1. total ECD: bullous keratopathy of the entire cornea

2. partial ECD: localised bullous keratopathy

3. minimal ECD: local stromal and/or epithelial oedema

The interval between implant operation date and first detection of incipient ECD in 64 out of 694 iris clip lens implant operations performed by BINKHORST, is shown in Fig. 3

| | | | | interval between implant operation and first detection of incipient ECD | | | | | |
| | | | | number per group | | | | | |
		number	%	$0-\frac{1}{4}$ year	$\frac{1}{4}$-1 years	1-4 years	>4 years	average (days)	range (days)
total	ECD	32	4.61	3	2	21	6	1088	0-2259
partial	ECD	10	1.44	0	1	5	4	1346	287-2240
minimal	ECD	22	3.17	2	6	7	7	1009	34-2830
total		64	9.22	5	9	33	17	1101	0-2830

Fig. 3. Interval between implant operation date and date of first detection of incipient ECD in 64 out of 694 iris clip lens implant operations performed by BINKHORST.

Fig. 3 shows that a post-operative interval of more than 4 years can occur before ECD becomes manifest and, moreover, that there is no correlation between the duration of this interval and the severity of the ECD that will ultimately develop.

The number of cases of ECD per 100 implant operations in the whole series, is shown in Fig. 4.

| | implant operation date no. 10, 200, etc. | number of eyes with | | |
		total ECD	partial ECD	minimal ECD
1st hundred	20- 9-62	8	–	1
2nd hundred	7-10-65	7	4	3
3rd hundred	29-11-67	8	3	10
4th hundred	14- 2-69	6	2	2
5th hundred	26-11-69	3	1	2
6th hundred	15- 1-71	–	–	4
last 94	9-12-71	–	–	–
total 694		32	10	22

Fig. 4. Distribution of ECD for every 100 cases amongst the 694 iris clip lens implant operations performed by BINKHORST.

It may be concluded that the incidence of ECD decreased only after 1-1-1969 when the loop length was reduced to 8 mm again. The length of the observation period is, of course, another important factor.

The distribution of *factors promoting ECD* in cases with total, partial and minimal ECD relative to the loop length used, is shown in Fig. 5.

loop length	number of eyes	number of eyes with ECD	endothelial touch	pre-operative FUCHS corneal dystrophy	serious operational and post-op. complications	no obvious reason
approx. 7 mm	96	8	1	1	5	1
approx. 8 mm	84	6	2	–	2	2
approx. 9 mm	214	40	24	8	7	1
8 mm	300	10	5	4	–	1
total	694	64	32	13	14	5

Fig. 5. Distribution of factors promoting ECD in cases with total, partial and minimal ECD, relative to the loop length used.

Remarkable is the fact that 24 out of 32 cases in the group showing endothelial touch originated from the 9 mm series. This stresses the importance of the loop length once again.

This is also demonstrated in Fig. 6 by the fact that the first 8 mm series shows a percentage of 7.14 for ECD, the 9 mm series of 18.69, and the second 8 mm series of 3.33.

The *consequences of ECD* are, in general, very grave indeed. In this series of 694 eyes, 38 eyes (5.48%) with total (32 x) or partial (6 x) ECD failed to regain a useful acuity. Four eyes with partial ECD have a visual acuity of only 0.4 to 0.7.

Up to a point one may say: when the number of dislocations increases, the number of cases developing ECD decrease, and the reverse. To avoid *both* complications in the use of the iris clip lens, has not been a complete success.

So much about the findings concerning dislocation and ECD in the series of BINKHORST himself, a series afflicted with all problems of pioneering work.

Let us now turn to dislocation and ECD in two other large series of iris clip lens implant operations, namely the series of WORST and that of the other 20 Dutch ophthalmologists who performed at least 8 individual Binkhorst lens implant operation up to 1-1-1972.

BINKHORST' percentages are high, but this is, of course, a result of his pioneering difficulties. In Fig. 2 and 4 we saw that his percentages dropped gradually in the latter hundreds of cases.

It may be concluded that in iris clip lens implant operations once the initial problems have been overcome, the percentage of dislocations would appear to be approximately 3, and of ECD approximately 2.5. Either of both percentages could, however, increase if the observation period were lengthened.

Now the percentages for these complications in cases fitted with another

	loop length	number of eyes	dislocation %	ECD %
11- 8-58 until 3- 8-62	approx. 7 mm	96	15.62	8.33
9- 8-62 until 3- 6-65	approx. 8 mm	84	23.81	7.14
10- 6-65 until 12-12-68	approx. 9 mm	214	2.34	18.69
9- 1-69 until 31-12-71	8 mm	300	4.53	3.33
11- 8-58 until 31-12-71		694	7.64	9.22

Fig. 6. Percentage of dislocation and ECD relative to the loop length series, in 694 iris clip lens implant operations performed by BINKHORST.

lens, namely the iridocapsular lens, will be considered. As you will know the iridocapsular lens does not have anterior loops, which would justify the expectation of a lower percentage of ECD.

	number of implant operations	average observation period (days)	dislocation		ECD (total or partial)	
			number of eyes	%	number of eyes	%
BINKHORST	694	772	53	7.64	42	6.05
WORST	485	245	13	2.68	11	2.27
20 other Dutch ophthalmologists	1011 (approx.)	314 (approx.)	30	2.97	27	2.67
total (approx.)	2190	443	96	4.38	80	3.65

Fig. 7. Comparison of BINKHORST, WORST and the 20 other Dutch ophthalmologists, relative to dislocation and ECD in approx. 2190 iris clip lens implant operations.

	number of implant operations	average observation period (days)	dislocation		ECD (total or partial)	
			number of eyes	%	number of eyes	%
BINKHORST	170	572	9	5.29	1	0.59
WORST	4	398	1		1	
17 other Dutch ophthalmologists	208 (approx.)	314 (approx.)	9	4.33	1	0.48
total (approx.)	382	430	19	4.97	3	0.79

Fig. 8. Comparison of BINKHORST, WORST and 17 other Dutch ophthalmologists, relative to dislocation and ECD in approximately 382 iridocapsular lens implant operations.

In this series 13 of the 19 dislocations occurred during the first two weeks after the operation.

The comparison of the percentages of dislocation and ECD is shown in Fig. 9.

	dislocation		ECD (total or partial)	
	iris clip lens	iridocapsular lens	iris clip lens	iridocapsular lens
BINKHORST	7.64	5.29	6.05	0.59
WORST	2.68		2.27	
22 other Dutch ophthalmologists	2.97	4.33	2.67	0.48
total	4.38	4.97	3.65	0.79

Fig. 9. Comparison of BINKHORST, WORST and 22 other Dutch ophthalmologists, of the percentage of dislocation and ECD in approximately 2190 iris clip lens implant operations and approximately 382 iridocapsular lens implant operations.

It may be concluded that the fixation of the iridocapsular lens causes more difficulties during the early post-operative period than that of the iris clip lens. On the other hand, the percentage of ECD is much lower for the iridocapsular lens than for the iris clip lens though this may possibly increase when the observation period has been extended.

The *big* difference between the percentage of ECD of the iris clip lens implants and that of the iridocapsular lens implants may not only be explained by the simple *presence* of the anterior loops in the iris clip lens, but also by their much greater *mobility* in cases operated on intracapsularly.

This greater mobility of the implant in intracapsular cases, if only for the antero-posterior movement effected by gravity, can be demonstrated by measuring the anterior chamber depth in the supine and the prone positions.

This was made possible by a construction, built according to instructions of Dr. BINKHORST, where a Haag-Streit slitlamp no. 900 with a depth measuring attachment II, attached to an examination table, could be directed downwards and upwards. This is shown in Fig. 10 and 11.

In Fig. 12 the average results of the measurements of the anterior chamber depth of 20 intracapsularly operated eyes are compared with those of 17 extracapsularly operated eyes.

The statistical conclusions drawn from these measurements are the following:

1. The average difference between the anterior chamber depth measured in the supine and prone positions, is in the intracapsularly operated eyes statistically significantly larger ($p < 0.05$) than in the extracapsularly operated eyes (0.24 against 0.12 mm).

2. The average anterior chamber depth measured in the supine position, is significantly smaller ($p < 0.05$) in the intracapsularly operated eyes than in the extracapsularly operated eyes (3.31 against 3.52 mm).

3. The average anterior chamber depth measured in the prone position, is also significantly smaller ($p < 0.05$) in the intracapsularly operated eyes than in the extracapsularly operated eyes (3.07 against 3.39 mm).

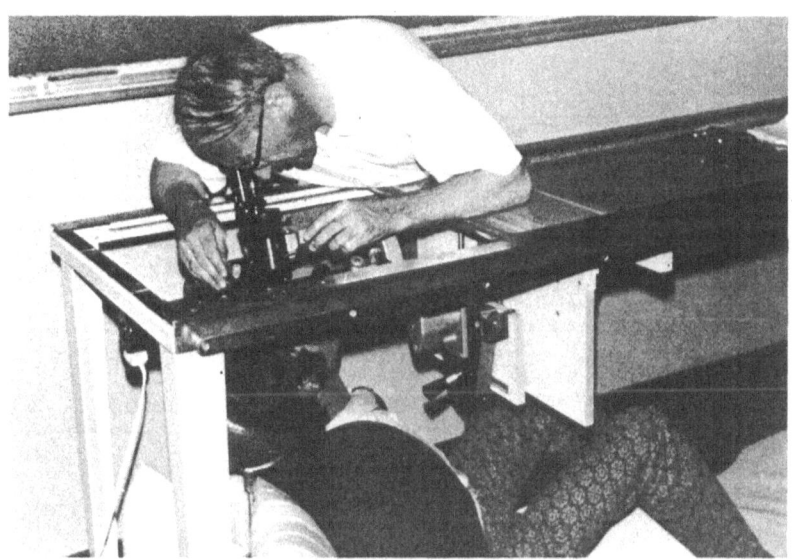

Fig. 10. The author measuring the anterior chamber depth with the patient's head supine

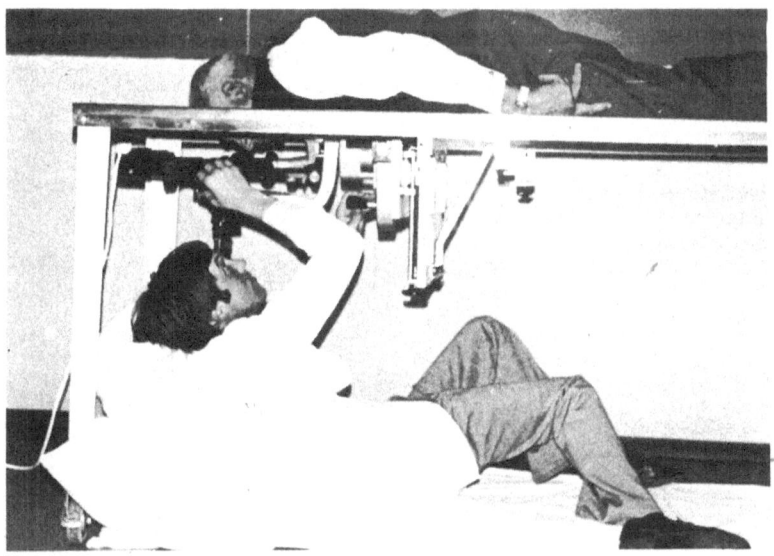

Fig. 11. L.H. LOONES measuring the anterior chamber depth with the patient's head prone.

It follows that in the prone position the implant approaches closer to the cornea in intracapsular cases than in extracapsular cases. Consequently, there is a bigger chance that ECD will occur due to endothelial touch by the anterior loops in intracapsular than in extracapsular cases.

Finally, this is also born out by the percentages of total and partial ECD in the iris clip lens series of BINKHORST .

21

| | anterior chamber depth (mm) | | |
	supine	prone	difference
20 intracapsular cases	3.31	3.07	0.24
17 extracapsular cases	3.52	3.39	0.12

Fig. 12. Results of the averaged measurements of the anterior chamber depth, with the patient's head supine or prone, in 20 intracapsular and 17 extracapsular cases of Binkhorst lens implants.

| | | dislocation | | ECD (total or partial) | |
	number	number	%	number	%
intracapsular cases	581	45	7.75	40	6.88
extracapsular cases	113	8	7.08	2	1.77
total	694	53	7.64	42	6.05

Fig. 13. Comparison of the percentages of dislocation and total or partial ECD in 581 intracapsular and 113 extracapsular cases of iris clip lens implant operations performed by BINKHORST.

In conclusion it may be said that BINKHORST lens implant operations are made safer by extracapsular extraction.

Author's address:
M.E. Nordlohne M.D.
Const. Huygenslaan 12
Vlissingen
The Netherlands

CURRENT STATUS OF INTRAOCULAR LENSES
IN THE UNITED STATES

NORMAN S. JAFFE

(Miami Beach)

When RIDLEY (1949) described an artificial lens and a technique for its introduction into the posterior chamber of the eye after an extracapsular extraction, it captured the imagination of ophthalmologists throughout the world. However, the subject has been and still remains one of the most controversial in all of ophthalmology. This comes as no surprise since the procedure makes an important modification in an operation which has proven one of the most successful in all of surgery. It differs in this respect from phaco-emulsification which is truly a modification of cataract surgery. Artificial lens implantations is a modification of the optical correction of aphakia.

In every lively scientific encounter there are those who present facts and those who offer opinions. It is distressing that many of the latter who have had little or no personal experience with the method and rare unaware of important recent modifications in the design of the lenses and the technique of their implantation, speak authoritatively on the·subject. This represents an injustice and tends to provide an unhealthy medicolegal arena for the further development of a useful procedure.

An attempt will be made to highlight previous attempts at substituting a plastic lenticulus for the crystalline lens and to summarize the current status of the procedure in the United States.

HISTORICAL

Because of uncertainties regarding the fixation of a Ridley lens within the posterior chamber, anterior chamber lenses were designed. When the latter presented a new set of problems (mainly late corneal edema), lenses were designed which depended entirely upon the iris for fixation. These lenses are located in the plane of the iris or slightly anterior. Thus, the evolution from one kind pseudophakos to another was based on complications which arose with earlier lenses. For example, the posterior chamber lens often caused uveitis by making contact with the ciliary body. In addition, it would occasionally dislocate into the vitreous itself since the thin posterior capsule of the crystalline lens could not consistently be depended upon to hold it in place.

The problem of secure fixation of the lens was solved with the introduction of anterior chamber lenses. However, corneal edema occurred in many of these eyes several years after insertion. This was presumed to be due to damage to angle structures, contact between the cornea and the lens, or due to reaction to the plastic lens. Unfortunately, this complication often arose after several years of satisfactory experience. However, marked improvements in the design of these implants have occurred, especially those introduced by CHOYCE.

A revival of enthusiasm for lens implant surgery arose when lenses were designed which were supported entirely by the iris. It was reasoned that such a lens was sufficiently separated from the cornea and angle structures that corneal edema would not occur. Although an iris supported lens was introduced by EPSTEIN of South Africa, C.D. BINKHORST supplied the major impetus for this enthusiasm.

CLASSIFICATION OF PSEUDOPHAKOS

The most convenient classification of artificial lenses is one based on their fixation within the eye.

1. Anterior chamber angle fixation

The haptic portion of the lens is held in place in the angle of the anterior chamber or externally. The optical portion is aligned with the pupillary aperture, anterior to the plane of the iris.
a. non-perforating rigid (STRAMPELLI, CHOYCE BOBERG-ANS) or non-perforating elastic (DANNHEIM). The haptic portion engages the angle of the anterior chamber (Figs. 1,2).

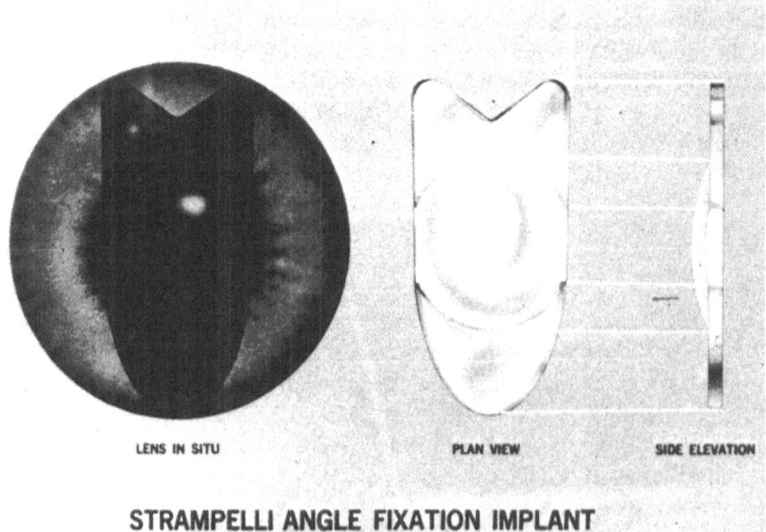

LENS IN SITU   PLAN VIEW   SIDE ELEVATION

STRAMPELLI ANGLE FIXATION IMPLANT

Fig. 1. Strampelli nonperforating, rigid anterior chamber angle implant. (From: JAFFE, N.S.: Cataract surgery and its complications, St. Louis, 1972, The C.V. Mosby Co.).

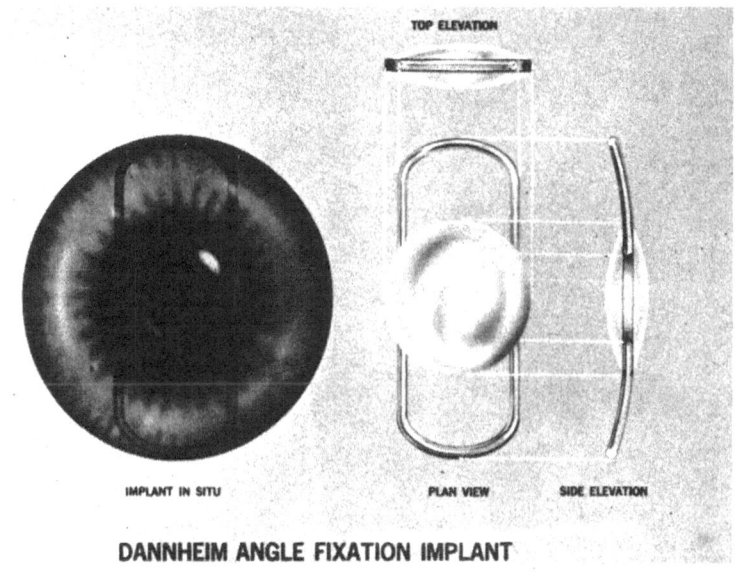

DANNHEIM ANGLE FIXATION IMPLANT

Fig. 2. Dannheim nonperforating, elastic anterior chamber implant. (From: JAFFE, N.S.: Cataract surgery and its complications, St. Louis, 1972, The C.V. Mosby Co.).

b. perforating (STRAMPELLI, CHOYCE). The haptic portion is brought out through the limbus and sutured in place on the sclera (Figs. 3,4).

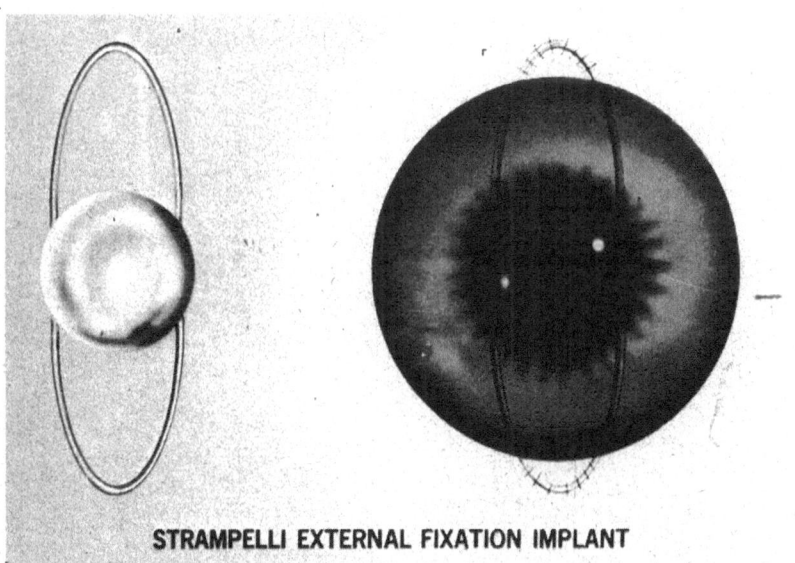

STRAMPELLI EXTERNAL FIXATION IMPLANT

Fig. 3. Strampelli perforating external fixation implant. (From: JAFFE, N.S.: Cataract surgery and its complications, St. Louis, 1972, The C.V. Mosby Co.).

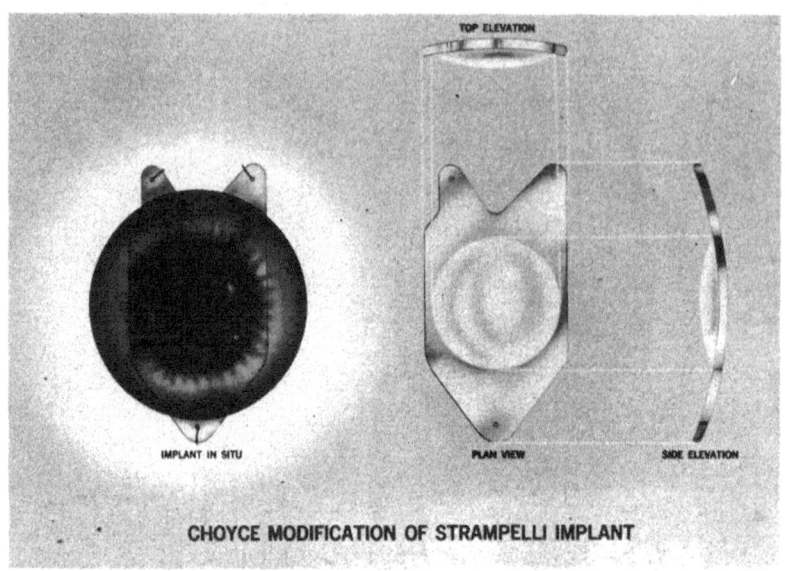

CHOYCE MODIFICATION OF STRAMPELLI IMPLANT

Fig. 4 Choyce perforating external fixation implant. (From' JAFFE, N S. Cataract surgery and its complications, St. Louis, 1972, The C.V Mosby Co.).

c. intrascleral (STRAMPELLI, BROWN). The haptic portion partially penetrates the limbus from within and is bent so as to lie within the slera.

2. Iris fixation (BINKHORST, EPSTEIN,
Iris-plane, FEDOROV) (Figs. 5,6)

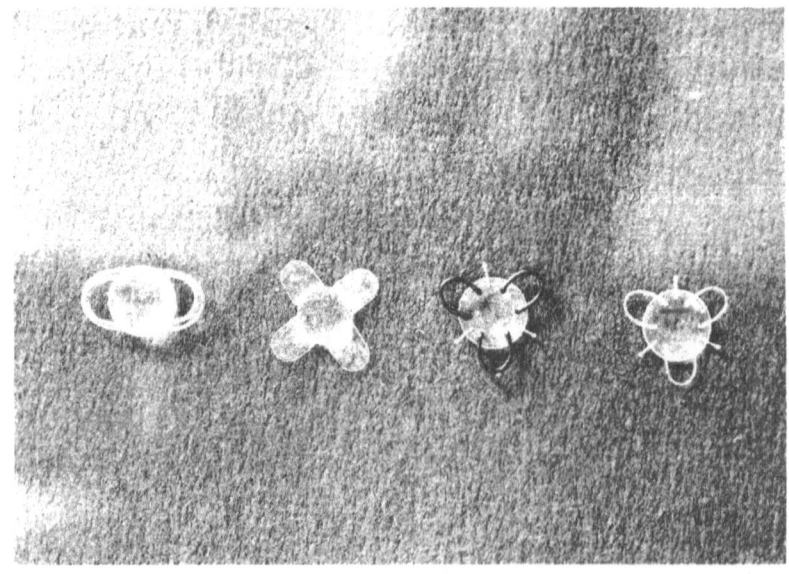

Fig 5. Iris-supported pseudophakoi. From left, Binkhorst iris clip lens, iris-plane lens, Fedorov lenses. (From JAFFE, N S. Cataract surgery and its complications, St Louis, 1972, The C V Mosby Co)

26

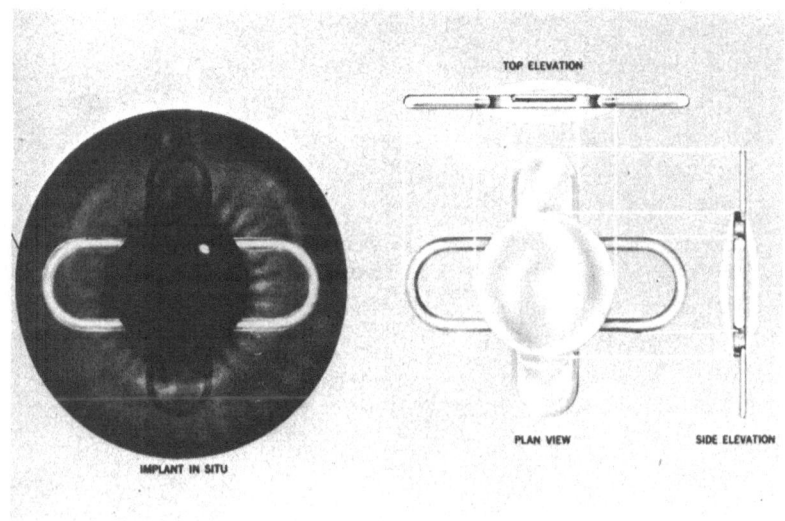

PLAN VIEW   SIDE ELEVATION

IMPLANT IN SITU

EPSTEIN IRIS FIXATION IMPLANT

Fig. 6. Epstein iris fixation implant. (From: JAFFE, N.S.: Cataract surgery and its complications, St. Louis, 1972, The C.V. Mosby Co.).

The haptic portion of the lens is chiefly supported by the iris. Some support is contributed by the anterior hyaloid membrane after an intracapsular lens extraction and the posterior capsule of the lens after an extracapsular extraction. The optical portion of the implant lies in the plane of the iris or just anterior or posterior to it. The haptic portion consists of loops which vary from fine to bulky. In the Binkhorst lens, the optical portion is made of poly-methylmethacrylate while the loops of the haptic portion consist of Dacron. The design of the haptic portion varies from the iris clip type to the iris cross type. In the former, there are 2 pairs of loops, an anterior and posterior. The iris fits between them. In the latter, there are 4 loops 90 degrees apart. Two opposite loops lie on the anterior surface of the iris while 2 lie against its posterior surface.

FEDOROV has designed a lens consisting of 3 loops which fit behind the iris and 3 small prongs between each loop which rest on the anterior surface of the iris.

The iris-plane lens is shaped like an airplane propeller. The haptic portion is solid. The shape of the pupil is square (4 mm.) with the Binkhorst and iris-plane lenses (Fig. 7) while it is hexagonal with the Fedorov lens (Fig. 8).

3. Irido-capsular fixation (RIDLEY (Fig. 9), BINKHORST, FEDOROV)

The lens is supported by the iris and the posterior capsule of the lens. Thus, an extracapsular cataract extraction is required. Ridley's original lens lay completely in the posterior chamber between the posterior surface of the iris and the posterior capsule of the lens. Since the major support was contributed by the lens capsule and since this must be extremely thin for

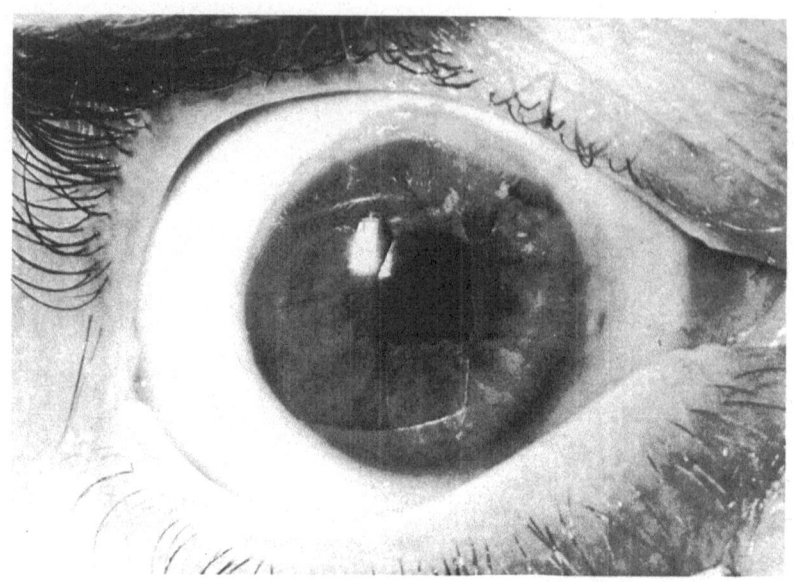

Fig. 7. Iris-plane lens. Solid haptic portions anterior to iris in vertical meridian. (From' JAFFE, N.S.: Cataract surgery and its complications, St. Louis, 1972, The C.V. Mosby Co.).

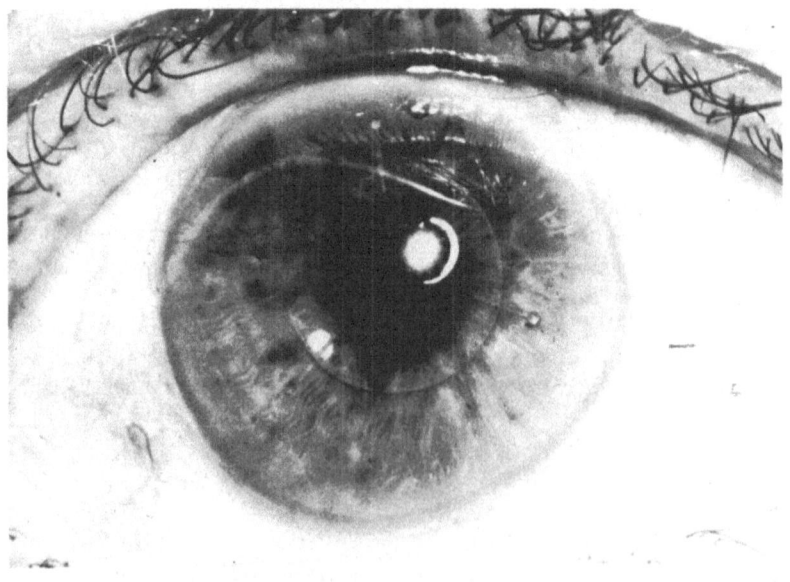

Fig. 8. Fedorov lens. Three supporting feet anterior to iris at 12, 4, and 8 o'clock. Nore hexagonal pupil. (From: JAFFE, N.S.: Cataract surgery and its complications. St. Louis, 1972, The C.V. Mosby Co.).

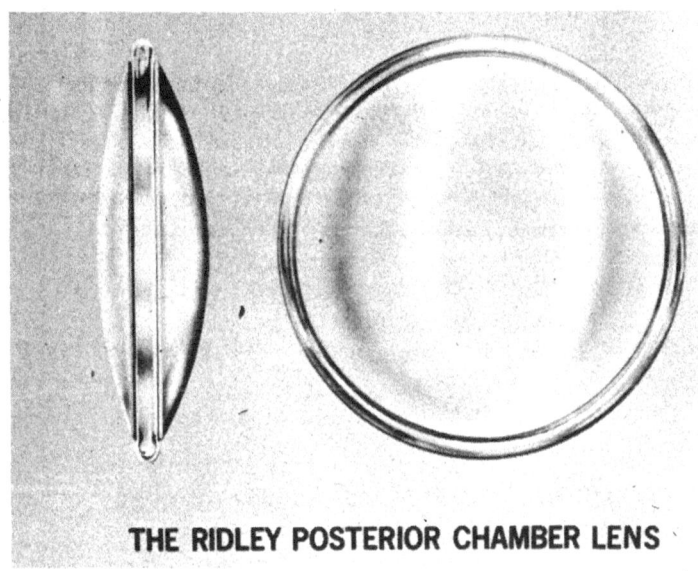

THE RIDLEY POSTERIOR CHAMBER LENS

Fig. 9. Ridley posterior chamber lens. (From: JAFFE, N.S.: Cataract surgery and its complications, St. Louis, 1972, The C.V. Mosby Co.).

optical reasons, the danger of dislocation of the implant was always great. Therefore, numerous modifications appeared which utilized the iris as well as the posterior capsule for fixation. The optical portion of the lens is located either in the anterior or posterior chamber. BINKHORST currently utilizes a pseudophakos with 2 posterior loops made of platinum-iridium. The loops adhere to the capsulo-cortical material while adherence of the iris is prevented. Therefore, it is really a capsular fixation type of implant.

4. Capsular fixation (FEDOROV)

This uncommonly used technique depends entirely on the posterior lens capsule for support.

ADVANTAGES AND INDICATIONS

One might question why an intraoccular lens is so superior to other methods of aphakic optical correction in view of the greater possibility of complications. These advantages are summarized as follows.

1. Visual

Vision most closely resembles that in the phakic eye than any other method. The lens rests close to the nodal point of the eye so that if the residual refractive error is minimal, most patients can manage without eyeglasses.

29

2. Refractive

It is not always possible to select a lens which will render the eye emmetropic. However, if the refractive error is known prior to the onset of cataract, a suitable power lens is available. The most exact method of selecting the proper lens is by computing it from the length of the eyeball (ultrasound), the depth of the anterior chamber and the corneal K reading. Most series of lens implantations reveal surprisingly little residual refractive error.

3. Perimetric

The visual field of the eye with an intraocular lens is the same as that of a normal phakic eye.

4. Aniseikonic

This technique provides the least amount of image size disparity of any method of correcting unilateral aphakia.

5. Psychological

The psychological stress suffered by so many aphakic patients in adapting to spectacles and contact lenses is completely eliminated by an intraocular lens. Patient acceptance is generally high.

The advantages of an iris-supported pseudophakos over one supported by the angle of the anterior chamber may be summarized as follows.
1. There is no contact with the anterior chamber angle, decreasing the incidence of iridocyclitis and corneal edema.
2. It is positioned much further away from the corneal endothelium, thereby lessening the incidence of corneal edema.
3. Exact centering by the iris sphincter muscle stabilizes the position of the implant.
4. The implant is less dependent on the configuration of the anterior chamber angle.
5. The implant is less dependent on the depth of the anterior chamber.

When intraocular lenses were first introduced, contact lenses were still in the early stages of their development. Today, contact lenses are much improved and patient tolerance is much higher. However, there are still a considerable number of elderly patients, nervous patients, and those with infirmaties such as hemiplegia, rheumatoid arthritis, athetosis, and Parkinsonism who cannot manage a contact lens.

An intraocular lens might be very valuable in preventing amblyopia and maintaining binocular vision in young children with a traumatic cataract. An eldery patient with a mature or advanced cataract in one eye and approximately 20/50 vision in the other eye often functions poorly since his vision in the sun and his reading vision are poor. Cataract extraction in only one eye with insertion of an intraocular lens will rehabilitate him, providing retinal function is normal. Another indication is the patient with disciform macular degeneration who develops an advanced cataract. Correction with spectacles is poor because his peripheral field (the only field he has) is reduced. His central vision is too poor to manage a contact lens.

SURGICAL TECHNIQUE

An intraocular lens should only be placed in an eye with a normal anterior segment. The lens may be inserted at the time of cataract surgery or subsequent to it. There are advantages to each. Performing a cataract extraction as an initial procedure provides an opportunity to learn the exact visual potential and refraction of the eye. If satisfactory, the implant may be inserted later. However, the advantage of performing a single procedure is obvious. My personal experience is limited to performing a cataract extraction and inserting the lens during the same procedure and it is also limited to pseudophakoi supported by the iris.

It is obvious that the condition of the vitreous immediately after the cataract extraction is vital for the successful insertion of an iris-supported pseudophakos. Since a portion of the haptic element of the lens must rest behind the iris, a bulge of vitreous is dangerous. Therefore, in addition to giving the patient a pre-operative hyperosmotic agent (glycerin or mannitol), I apply at least 7 minutes of digital pressure, perform a liberal lateral canthothomy, and delay the cataract incision until the Schiotz tonometer registers 15 scale units or more using a 5.5 gm. weight. Although some surgeons insert the lens through the closed cornea, I prefer to place it under direct observation, with the cornea retracted. This requires a large incision, at least 180 degrees in amplitude. If the vitreous is well retracted, the iris falls back with it. To facilitate insertion of the lens, balanced salt solution is instilled in the eye. This floats the iris up away from the vitreous. The iris-plane lens with which I have had my greatest experience, is grasped at the tip of one of the haptic supports. The nasal support is inserted under the iris and by retracting the nasal portion of the iris, sufficient clearance is obtained to permit placement of the temporal support behind the temporal part of the iris. The vertical supports are placed anterior to the iris. If preferred by the surgeon, the vertical supports may be placed behind the iris and the horizontal supports anterior to it.

If the vitreous bulges after the cataract is extracted, a 22 gauge needle is inserted through a peripheral iridectomy and retrovitreal fluid is aspirated. This reduces the vitreous bulge and makes implantation easier.

PERSONAL EXPERIENCE

The results of all cases of artificial lens implantation performed in the Miami community during the past 6 years are currently being tabulated. Therefore, I will emphasize only a few points from my own personal experience.

As in Holland, corneal edema does not represent a significant problem. The two main complications encountered are cystoid macular edema and intraocular lens membranes. In most instances, the diagnosis of the former is possible with biomicroscopy and a Hruby lens. Fluorescein angiography is also possible through the relatively undilatable pupil. I have the impression, but no statistical evidence at this time, that cystoid macular edema is more common than after routine cataract extraction and when it occurs it tends to persist longer. Intraocular lens membranes are more frequent than with the pseudophakoi used in Holland. This may be due to the closer proximity of the optical portion of the pseudophakos to the vitreous face. Adhesions of the lens to the anterior hyaloid membrane may result in opaque condensations on the back of the pseudophakos.

I have had a poor experience in relatively young patients with senile cataract compared to the older age group. Very few young patients had pseudophakos implantations in the Miami area and these only early in our series. The following was encountered in patients under 60 years of age. There were 13 eyes in 12 patients. It was necessary to remove the implant in 5 of 13 eyes. This was due to persistent or recurrent iritis, with or without secondary glaucoma and corneal edema. Four of these 5 patients had routine cataract extraction in the opposite eye without complications. All attained 20/20-20/25 visual acuity. Five of the 13 eyes showed persistent cystoid macular edema. Two of the 5 had routine cataract extraction in the opposite eye with no cystoid macular edema. One should be wary of young patients with senile cataract, especially those which are unilateral. In my view, a cataract in a young patient represents something wrong in a sick eye.

It is surprising how well the ocular tissues tolerate a pseudophakos in uncomplicated cases (Fig. 10). An effort should be made to obtain as many postmortem pseudophakic eyes as possible for histologic examination.

Undoubtedly newer and better lenses will be designed in the future. However, at this time the procedure of lens implantation plays an important role in the rehabilitation of many patients with disabling cataracts.

CURRENT APPROACH

A brisk, often heated dialogue has ensued during the past seven years between lens implant surgeons and their critics. The disastrous results of anterior chamber lenses in the early and middle 1950's, the fear that the delicate internal structure of an eye cannot tolerate the presence of a large foreign body, and the requirement for excellent surgical technique in implanting an artificial lens have been genuine sources of concern. Critics reasoned that there would occur an epidemic of lens implantations before adequate time trials of current techniques could be evaluated. They further stated that less qualified surgeons or those who did not favor the procedure would be forced into performing lens implantations as a result of economic pressures generated by their colleagues who favor the operation.

Lens implant surgeons in the Miami community have taken a unique approach to assemble data which will be truly meaningful in determining the safety and value of the procedure. A Pseudophakos Registry was organized so that data could be kept on every lens implantation (without exception) performed. Every patient was examined annually by ophthalmologists most of whom do not perform the operation and the data were recorded. Each year in June, the results have been reported. It is to the credit of the participating surgeons that a two year moratorium on lens implantations was declared on Oct. 1, 1969 since it was felt that a sufficient number of eyes

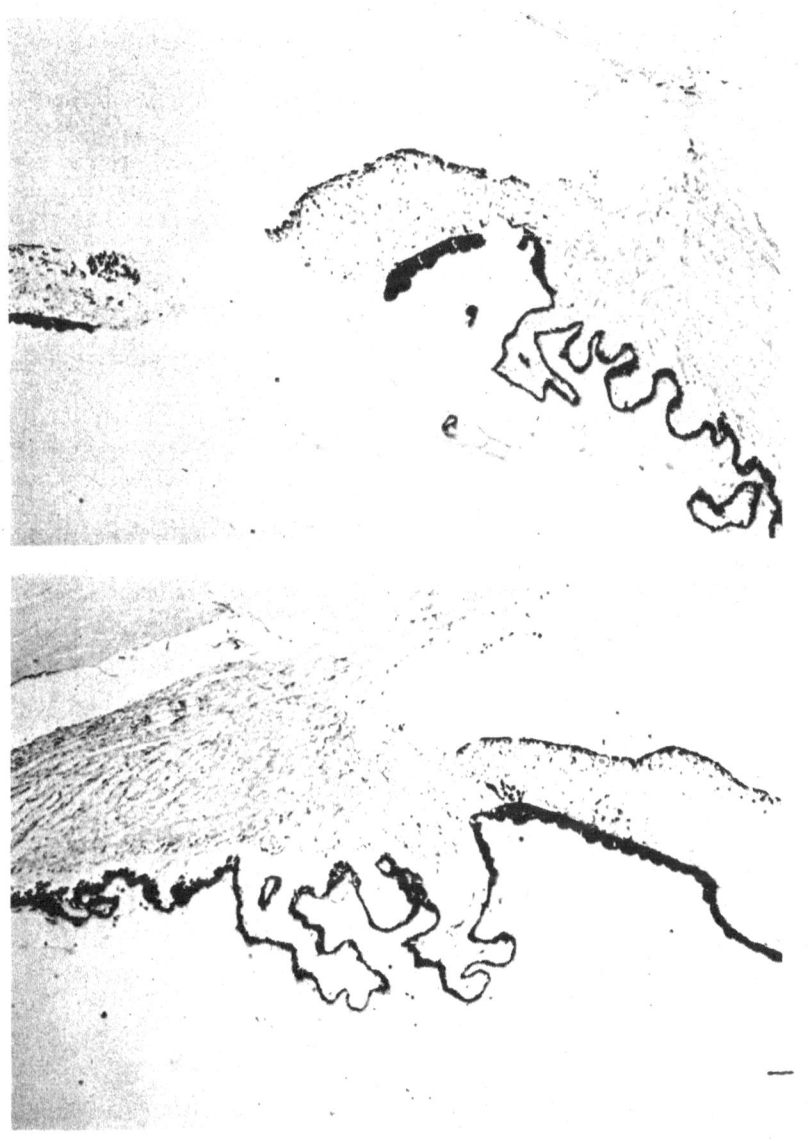

Fig. 10. Postmortem eye of a 63-year-old male who died 7 months after insertion of an iris-plane lens. A, Upper angle in area of iridectomy. B, Lower angle of same eye. Note remarkable lack of inflammation. (From: JAFFE, N.S.: Cataract surgery and its complications, St. Louis, 1972, The C.V. Mosby Co.).

(243) operated upon before that date were available for a meaningful study. It was stated that if the eyes continued to fare well, the moratorium would be lifted on Oct. 1, 1971. The June, 1971 report was sufficiently encouraging to warrant a resumption of the procedure. However, the following strict guidelines were suggested. It is emphasized that this is a voluntary

restriction agreed upon in the Miami community and is not intended to reflect unfavorably on surgical indications accepted by ophthalmologists in other communities.

1. Lens implantations were restricted to patients over 70 years of age. This was later changed to 67 years of age.

2. A pseudophakos could not be placed in the second eye of a patient until a five year successful interval has elapsed since lens implantation in the first eye. This was later changed to four years. If the patient is over 80 years of age, this interval is reduced to one year.

3. Exceptions may consist of physically or mentally handicapped patients (hemiplegics, arthritics, tremors, macular degeneration, etc.). A panel of three ophthalmologists determines the validity of the exception.

4. All artificial lens implantations must be registered with the Pseudophakos Registry.

5. An annual survey of all cases is to be continued.

6. In order to reduce economic pressure on other ophthalmologists in the community, each surgeon is restricted to a specific number of lens implantations per year.

7. These guidelines may be altered according to the results of the annual survey.

Thus, the Miami community has taken cognizance of criticism of artificial lens implantations but it has taken a unique step as a community to determine the true role of the procedure in cataract surgery.

SOME METHODICAL ASPECTS OF THE IMPLANTATION OF BINKHORST LENSES

J. DRAEGER

(Bremen)

Abstracted and translated by A.TH.M. VAN BALEN

In certain phases of the implantation operation microsurgical equipment should be used.

Pedal-switch operated focussing and zooming as well as remote control of lateral movements of the operation table are indispensable for surgery under the microscope.

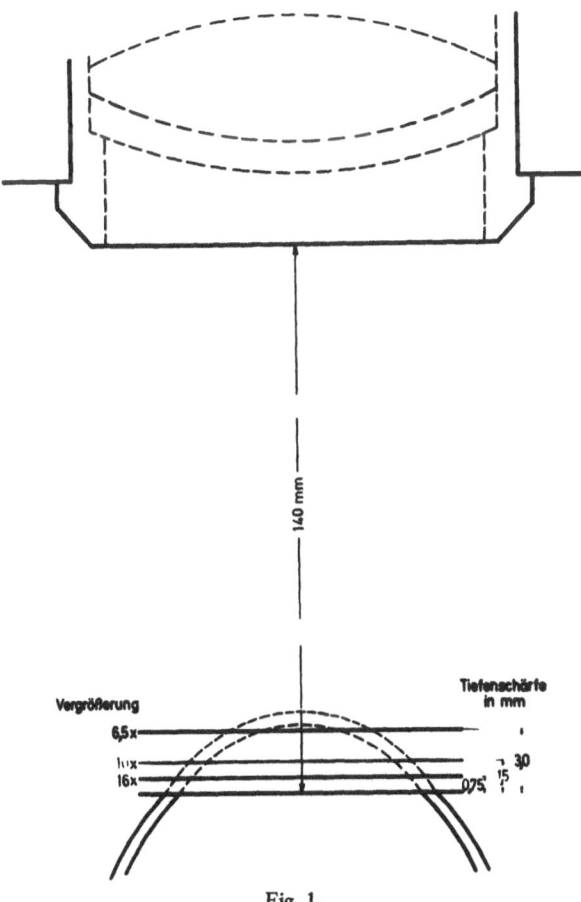

Fig. 1.

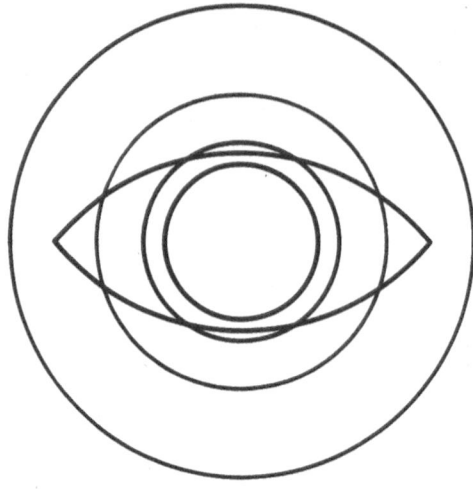
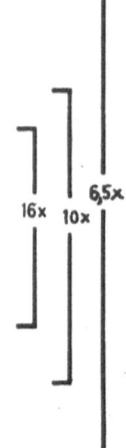

Fig. 2.

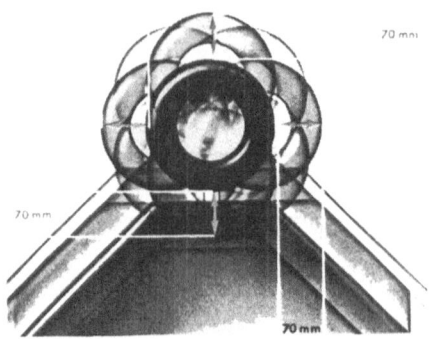

Fig. 3.

For the implantation of an artificial lens a normal reacting pupil is preferred. For this reason, cryoextraction seems to be less suitable. Apart from forceps extraction the erisophake is recommended.

The suction apparatus is completely pedal controlled. Both hands are free for the actual extraction.

In the first stage of the implantation operation a vertical movement of the forceps holding the Binkhorst lens is made. The microscope has to follow this movement. For the insertion of the posterior loops between the anterior vitreous membrane and the iris, a sufficient magnification is necessary. While increasing the magnification, the focal depth will decrease. Remote controlled focussing compensates for this without the necessity for the surgeon to take his hands from the field of operation.

Figure 1 illustrates the influence of the magnification on the depth of focus. Illumination is a crucial point in microsurgical work. The newly designed operation microscope has been fitted with a handle for switching over from oblique to coaxial illumination. Moreover the angle of slitlamp illumination is variable and the slit can be rotated and decentrated. All technical functions can be controlled from the surgeon's chair.

Figure 2 gives the visual field of the surgeon in relation to the magnification used. The lateral movement of the operation table may be used to compensate for the small field, as is the case with the cross table of a microscope.

Figure 3 shows this for the highest magnification available (16x). In this paper only methodical refinements of microsurgery have been discussed. Reporting the results of personally performed implantations would be like 'carrying owls to Athens'. Successfully implanted patients are among the most grateful and this is a reason for thanking Dr. BINKHORST.

Author's address:
J. Draeger
Eye Clinic
Zentrall-Krankenhaus
Bremen
B.R.D.

THE AUTHOR'S TECHNIQUE FOR LENS
IMPLANTATION (IRIS 'MEDALLION' LENS)

J.G.F. WORST

(Haren, Gr.)

Over a period of 4 years some 1500 lensimplantations have been performed with the socalled iris medallion lens (Fig. 1A, 1B).

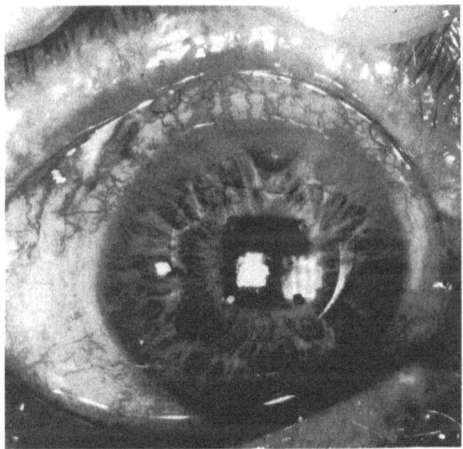

Fig. 1A.

This lens is a pupil supported lens, based on the iris clip lens principle of BINKHORST. The only essential modification has been its additional fixation to the iris by means of a Perlon suture (Fig. 2).

A further element characteristic of this lens is the absence of anterior loops, which have been replaced by an excentric haptic part. The function of this haptic part, and the sutures passed through it, is to maintain the lens in contact with the upper pupillary border, in order to prevent luxation. Fig. 3 shows the typical position of the sutured iris medallion lens in a dilated pupil. This procedure seemed in no need of further modification, until it was noted that in some case the Perlon suture failed. This had no consequences on the fixation of the lens, but entailed the risk of contact of the loose suture with the endothelium. In cases of suture failure it may therefore be necessary to remove it.

Description of the technique for iris medallion lens suture removal falls outside the scope of this part of the paper, but will be treated in: 'Pitfalls and Complications of Lensimplantation' (in preparation). This procedure

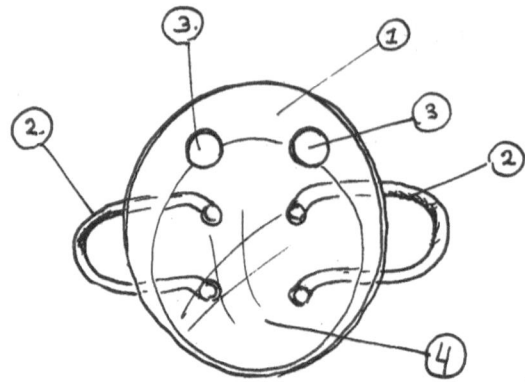

Fig.1B IRIS MEDALLION LENS ("MARK I")
A LENS WITH AN EXCENTRIC HAPTIC FLANGE (1)
TWO POSTERIOR LOOPS (2)
TWO HOLES FOR SUTURE PASSAGE (3)
A CENTRAL OPTICAL PART
OF 20 DIOPTERS (4)

Fig. 1B.

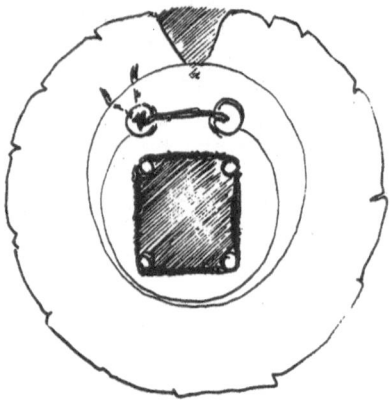

Fig.2. IRIS MEDALLION LENS, SUTURED TO
THE IRIS WITH A PERLON STITCH.

Fig. 2.

for suture removal proved a rapid, safe and effective method.

The reasons for suture failure were twofold:

1. Some sutures simply 'chafed' through on the edge of the lens holes because of the continuous movement of the iris to light. This mechanical failure is therefore due to 'plastic fatigue'.

2. Some sutures were biochemically absorbed. This absorption started with

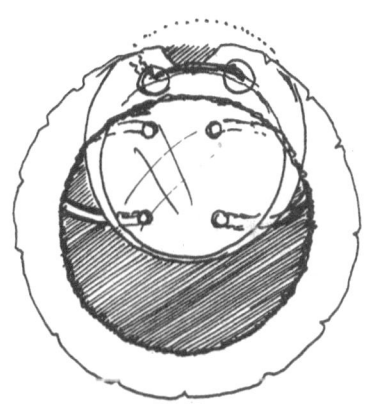

Fig. 3A IRIS MEDALLION LENS. DILATED PUPIL.
LENS FIXATION IS BASED ON
DISPLACEMENT OF THE LENS, WHICH
PREVENTS LUXATION, BY MAINTAINING
POSTERIOR LOOPS IN THE POSTERIOR
CHAMBER

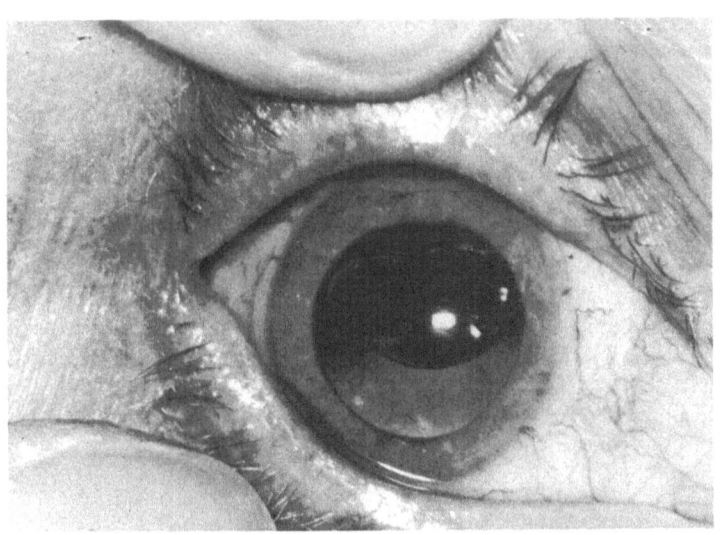

a discoloration of the black suture, followed by local swelling and finally by a progressive disappearance.

The same phenomenon has been remarked by German investigators (DODEN, personal communications).

Usually such absorption started at the free ends of the suture and not only on the part embedded in iris tissue. It seems likely therefore that some enzymatic action of the aqueous humour has been active in suture absorption.

The question why only some 1% of cases showed this phenomenon could at first not be solved. It proved however, that most of the cases showing this phenomenon had been operated in a circumscribed period of time. It seemed safe therefore to assume that a degraded batch of Perlon had been used during that period. It was further assumed that overtreatment with Gamma irridation could be the initial cause of degradation. There is no doubt now that this is indeed the most likely explanation, for the following reasons:

1 Sutures, which have been purposedly overexposed to an overdose of Gamma sterilizing irridation by repeated resterilization loose their mechanical strength and finally disintegrate in the package. (P.V.C. package, not nylon).

2. Metal sutures (stainless steel) overexposed in the same sterilizing process as the Perlon sutures will disintegrate in the package as well, if packed in P.V.C.

If a biochemical factor alone were involved there should be a much higher percentage of suture failures. In fact, sutures put in 6 years ago show no tendency to absorption or other failures. These sutures were sterilised by ethylene oxide, instead of by Gamma irradiation.

Nevertheless, the author's procedure of suturing artificial lenses to the iris showed a serious potential risk, for a small minority of patients.

The author has therefore designed a new technique for iris fixation of the iris medallion lens based on the original principle but using stainless steel in stead of Perlon as a suturing material.

With truely non absorbable artificial filaments the suturing technique can be safely continued. At the moment of writing the steel suture has been applied to 25 cases.

There are indications that the steel suture technique is safer than the Perlon procedure and will therefore in the course of time replace the author's Perlon iris stitch for irismedallion and other intraocular lens fixation. Other methods of fixation are now in use as well. See: 'Lens design'.

Except for the technique of the stainless steel iris suture no major modification has appeared in the author's technique for lens implantation of the iris medallion lens. It seems safe therefore to give a detailed description of what is now considered a standard procedure. The surgical method is essentially a 'preparative' one.

Draping of the surgical field.

A full covering of the eyelids and eyelashes is even more important than in conventional cataract surgery, as contamination may occur when the artificial lens touches extraocular structures. The draping is performed with a series of 6 'Steridrape' strips, cut from a 'Steridrape' packet (see Fig. 4).

Four strips are stuck to the eyelids in a diamondshaped configuration. The eyelashes are carefully folded backwards under the drapes, and should not be cut (Fig. 5).

Care must be taken to apply these strips in a progressive manner in order to prevent the formation of 'pockets' under the drape. Washing fluids tend

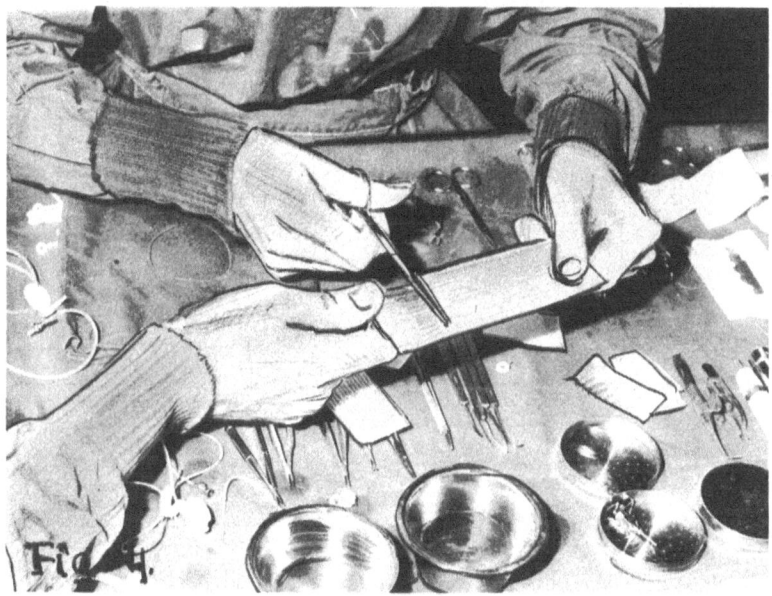

Fig. 4.

to collect in these 'pockets' and will be washed intraocularly at a later stage. After applying the four strips in a diamond shaped figure the author's malleable disposable lidholder (Fig. 6) is applied over the drape. For a proper fixation of these lidholders a special procedure fixing the head to the operating table is essential. This type of three point bandage support for head fixation is shown in Fig. 7. It is the vertical (cranial) strip, which immobilizes the frontal muscle, which is the most essential part of the fixation procedure (Fig. 8).

In case of general anesthesia the upper and lower eyelids are drawn away with the author's lid retractors. In case of local anesthesia it may be advisable to retract only the upper eyelid.

If the lower lidholder is also applied, movement of the facial muscles may cause dangerous vertical movements of this lidholder. These lidholders are individually adjustable and as they are not joined by a spring there are no vectorial forces leading to increased intraocular pressure, when the spreading becomes too forcible. The individual adjustment to the eyelid configuration and orbital rim further makes possible an asymmetric retraction, with preference for the upper eyelid. This exposes the surgical area more effectively. There are further no screws or other obstacles in this lidholder, a point of some importance in lens implantation as the intraocular sutures can not become ensnared.

After application of the four strips the author's suction irrigation system (Fig. 9) must be attached to the surgical field. This suction irrigation system is a procedure for maintaining complete corneal clarity and also serves for washing away any potential contaminants. This system consists of an irrigating device and a suction canula (see Fig. 9). The suction canula should be placed in the nasal angle and is than fixed with the fifth Steridrape strip.

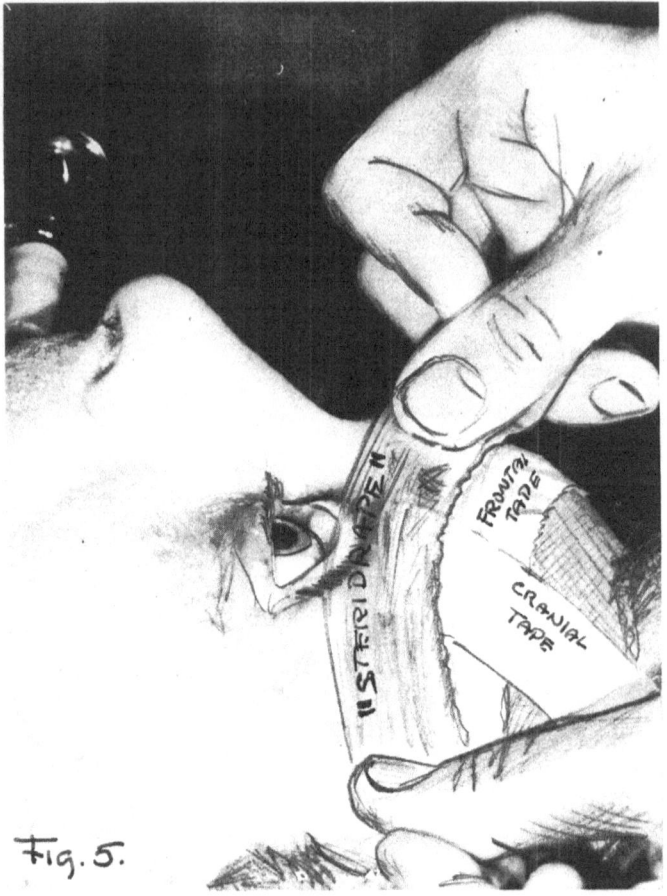

Fig. 5.

The sixth Steridrape strip is now folded backwards on itself so as to make both sides adhesive. This double adhesive strip is placed over the forehead. It serves for full immobilization of the final covering drape.

The irrigating device can now be clamped to the edge of the covering drape. The aspiration and the irrigation device have been made of the same malleable aluminium as the lidholders and are therefore individually adjustable. In case a microscope is used DREWS system for placement of the continuous drip is preferable: The drip is fastened to the microscope between the objectives (DREWS, personal communication). The irrigation device is connected to an intravenous drip bottle containing balanced salt solution. A filter should be included in the system as most commercial saline solutions, though sterile, are not absolutely particle free. Foreign body free technique is an essential part of the surgical procedure for lens-implantation. A freedom of particles is obtained by systematic filtering of all fluids and all air used around and in the eye. Fluid cleaning is obtained by means of Millipore filters. The air is made particle free by means of a special air flow system. (see Fig. 7).

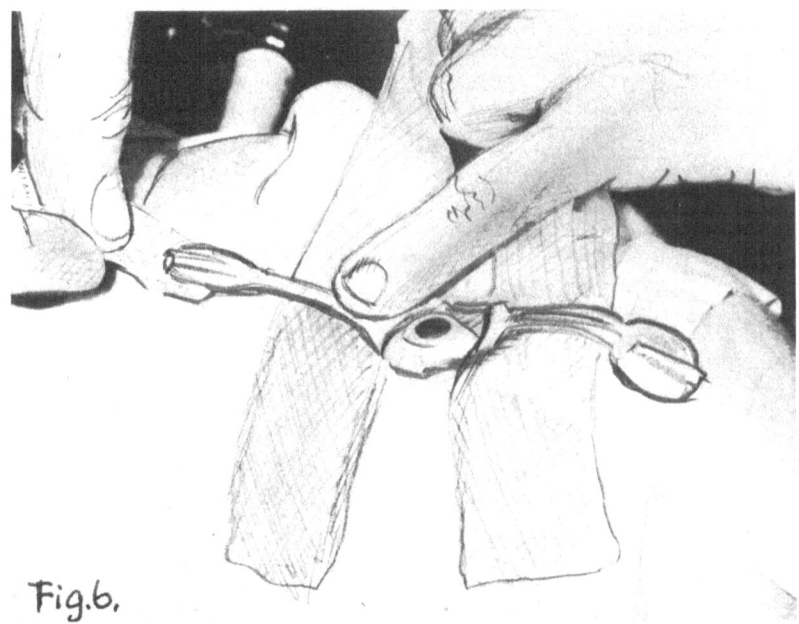

Fig. 6.

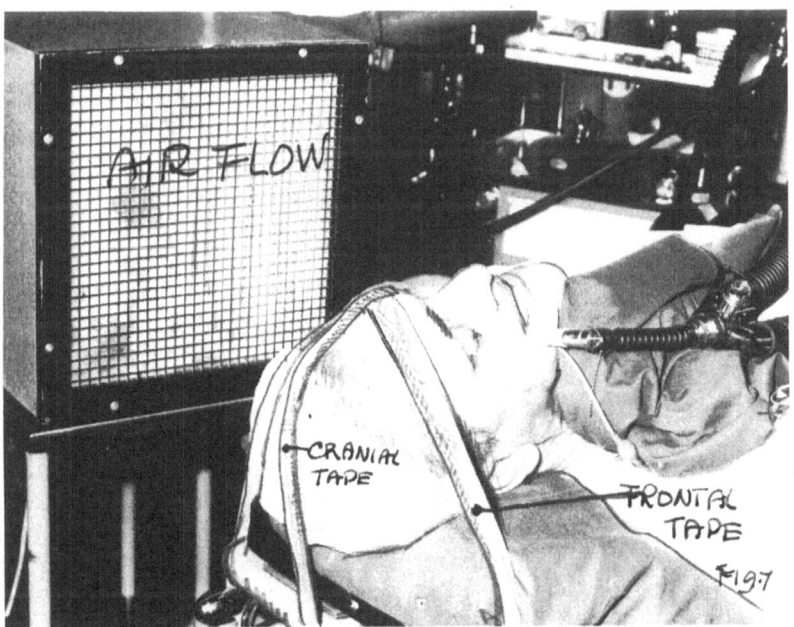

Fig. 7.

These fluid and air filtering systems are of paramount importance and disregard of this rule may lead to seriously inflamed eyes. The tendency to ascribe late iritis to the presence of the lens as such is a common error. In

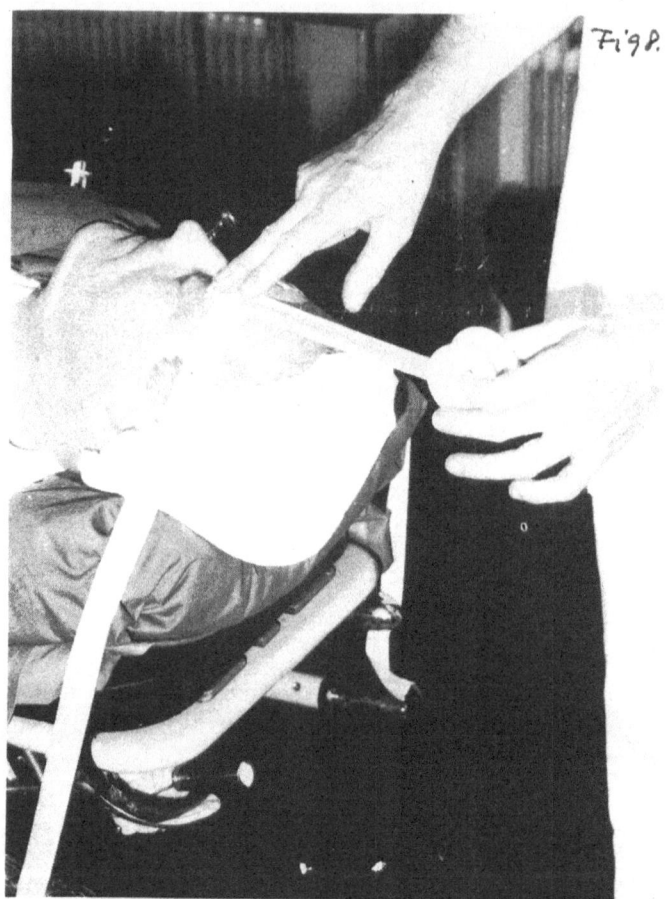

Fig. 8.

fact most late postoperative irritations are due to bacterial or biochemical contaminants, in stead of the lens itself.

Usually some form of lint or other foreign body is the cause of irritation. Strict observance of the contamination free techniques as mentioned in this paper are therefore essential. It is our experience from teaching the procedure in various courses that the purely surgical techniques are adopted but that the more circumstantial precautions are omitted as the specialized equipment is not available right away.

Note: To start the irrigation system one should put some pressure on the intravenous drip system as the resistance in the canula leading to the irrigator is too high to expel air by hydrostatic pressure only. Once the system has started to drip, hydrostatic pressure of some 60 cm. water is sufficient to maintain a continuous drip.

FLIERINGA'S RING (Fig. 10)

For a safe insertion of any intraocular lens the position of the iris-lens

46

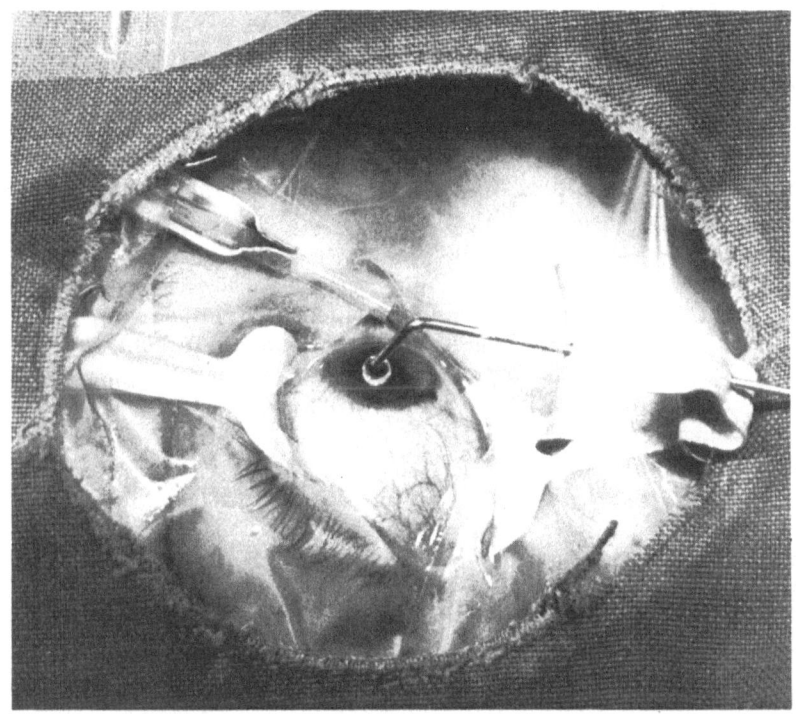

Fig. 9.

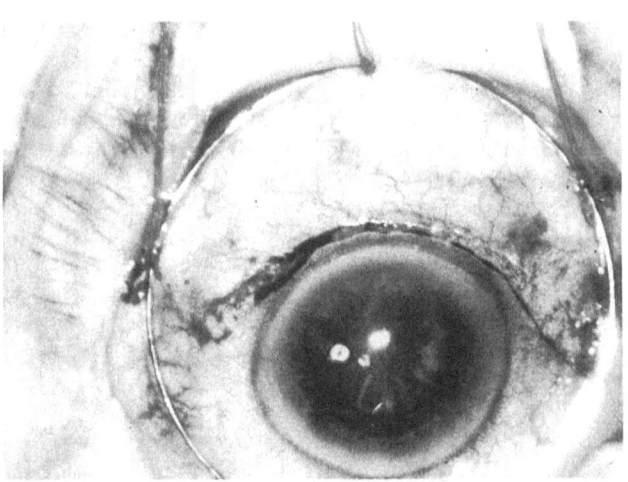

Fig. 10.

diafragm is of considerable importance.

Only when the intraocular pressure behind this diafragm is sufficiently low, the diafragm will remain in the appropriate flat position. Any pressure from the vitreous cavity results in an unpleasant forward bulge. This forward presentation of the iris-lens diafragm may already be an indication that

47

lensimplantation will not be possible. If after lens extraction the vitreous surface presents itself in a menacing convex manner all plans to perform a lens implantation should be abandoned, unless one is highly experienced in the procedure. Various technical measures are available to cope with presenting vitreous body or even manifest vitreous loss. This paper is concerned with routine lens implantation only and special problems will be subject of a later communication. (Pitfalls and Complications of Lens Implantation, in preparation).

The author has found that the use of Flieringa's ring in combination with anesthesia administered by a professionally skilled anesthesist, who is familiar with the problems of lens implantation is the most effective way to maintain the vitreous surface in its proper flat position. It should be noted that also a negative vitreous problem' may be created, in which the vitreous body and the iris fall backwards in the vitreous cavity. For the management of this 'complication' see also: Pitfalls and Complications of Lens Implantation (in preparation).

The relation between the preoperative intraocular pressure and the postoperative appearance of the vitreous membrane is an interesting matter, which deserves some attention here. It is usually claimed that a low preoperative pressure is favourable for the final position of the lens-iris diafragm. In order to produce the lowest possible pressures many author's advocate the use of mannitol or related dehydrating agents. Diamox is further given routinely. In our experience however there is no strict relation between the initial intraocular pressure and the behaviour of the vitreous body during surgery unless the pressure is caused by external factors. The idea that the internal pressure must be the lowest possible in order to maintain the intravitreal pressure at the lowest possible level is a fallacy. It has correctly been said that the best way to produce zero intraocular pressure is simply to open the anterior chamber with an incision.

As an example of the absence of a relation between the intraocular pressure and the vitreous behaviour during surgery one can demonstrate the cases of glaucoma in which lens extraction is performed. Even with pressures between 25 and 30, which have failed to respond to treatment, the intraocular procedure usually runs without problems and in these glaucoma cases the vitreous body tends to fall backwards in stead of presenting itself in the pupil.

If the initial pressure had any bearing on the vitreous behaviour one would expect frequent problems with the vitreous body in case of glaucoma. It is our thesis that virtually all vitreous presentation is caused by external pressure factors.

The worst factor in this respect is pressure from local anesthetics or muscle pressure due to insufficient local or general anesthesia. The intraocular pressure as such bears no relation to the intravitreal pressures, which are the main cause of vitreous presentation.

Truely intravitreal pressures, which are fortunately rare, are due to incipient and abortive choroidal hemorrhage. The vast majority of cases however, which show increased vitreous pressure are due to external scleral pressure factors. To relieve this external pressure, f.i. simple collaps of the sclera, or muscle- and eyelid pressure, Flieringa's ring has proved a most effective mechanical preventive procedure.

In my experience this procedure is more effective than external massage or intravenous mannitol infusion together.

It is further far less agressive on the general wellbeing of the patient. It should be noted however, that the application of Flieringa's ring is a surgical procedure in its own right and should be taught carefully before it is adopted.

THE TECHNIQUE OF FLIERINGA'S RING

1. The conjunctiva may be opened before applying the ring. This particularly facilitates the placement of the two lateral stitches. However, there is no difference in the surgical technique of Flieringa's ring whether the conjunctiva is opened or kept intact. (Fig. 10).

2. The choice of the size of the ring.

The largest ring must be chosen, which one can still insert easily between the eyelids. This may therefore be a small ring when the palpebral aperture is narrow. In case of a large myopic eye there is usually a large palpebral aperture as well and a 22 or 23 mm. ring is normal. It is the general tendency to use too small a ring. Rings sizes vary between 18 and 23 mm.

The first stitch is placed with a special roundtipped needle. Cutting needles of any sort are wrong. These may perforate inadvertently through local sclerectasias, and episcleral vessels may be ruptured causing sub-conjunctival hemorrhages. The sutures attached to the needle should be 6-0.

The original suture as used by Flieringa is green Jenilene ('mersilene silk').

A point of technical interest is the preparation of the needle-suture com bination. These are fastened to the so called Flieringa's 'ring book'. Each suture should be double and 25 cm long, but one of the suture ends should be made some 3 cm longer.

This difference in length is a simple but important technical detail. Sutures of the type as shown in Fig. 11a are incorrect. Sutures of the type of Fig. 11b are correct.

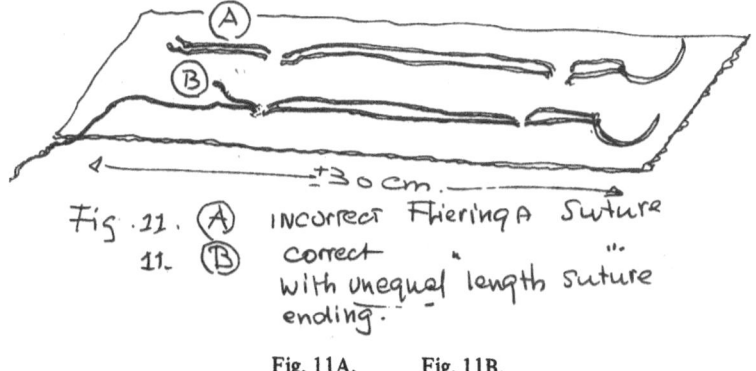

Fig. 11A.   Fig. 11B.

If the 11a suture is used there is a chance of pulling the suture from the needle when passing the long suture through the sclera. Each stitch must be placed in a sclero-corneal direction and little or no forceps fixation of the globe should be used.

The natural tendency of the round tipped needle to find the episcleral tissues is sufficient to make the correct episcleral bite.

The first stitch is placed over the superior rectus area at ± 6 mm. from the limbus. This results in an excentric position of the ring. The excentric position of the ring is an essential point of Flieringa's ring technique, which is often forgotten (Fig. 10).

The second stitch is placed at 6 o'clock area at the point of contact of the ring with the eye.

This varies with the size of the eye and of the ring in individual cases.

The third and fourth stitch are placed over the upper edges of the external and internal rectus muscles.

The three upper sutures are left long, and are joined in one knot. This knot is clamped to the drape over the forehead. The three upper sutures serve also as a superior rectus bridle. With some experience the placement of a Flieringa ring takes 2 to 3 minutes.

This technique uses four stitches only. The original technique of FLIE-RINGA indicates eight sutures. HENKES (personal communications) uses 6 sutures. We believe the 4 sutures to be sufficient. As during lens implantation changes of position of the eye may be necessary, the ring is a very useful adjunct to put the eye in the required position without increasing the intra-vitreal pressure.

The excentric position of the ring makes it possible to place the surgical area and not the corneal apex in the center of the operative field.

Flieringa's ring is a very effective way of obtaining maximum surgical exposure without undue external pressures.

The clamping of the ring sutures produces an extremely effective stabilization of the eye, which facilitates 'preparative' surgical techniques like the making of a preliminary half depth corneo-scleral section.

It has been stated that Flieringa's ring is often superfluous. This is correct. But as it is impossible to predict when the ring will be effective in preventing vitreous loss it should, in the author's opinion, always be applied.

An instruction film on the use of Flieringa's ring can be made available by the author. The autor has also designed a special needle-suture combination for Flieringa's ring surgery (not illustrated).

THE CONJUNCTIVAL SECTION (Fig. 12)

A small snip parallel to and at about 1mm from the limbus is made with sharp scissors at the 12 o'clock position. The dissection is carried down to the bare sclera. Starting from this local dissection large horizontal snips are made through all layers. This results in a conjunctival section, which diverges from the corneal scleral limbus and is only tangential to it at the 12 o'clock area. The section should extend to the semilunar fold in the medial angle and to the lateral canthus on the temporal side.

The subconjunctival tissues are now dissected bluntly towards the 3 and 9 o'clock positions of the limbal area. The results will be that combined limbal based and fornix based flaps have been made. The limbal based areas

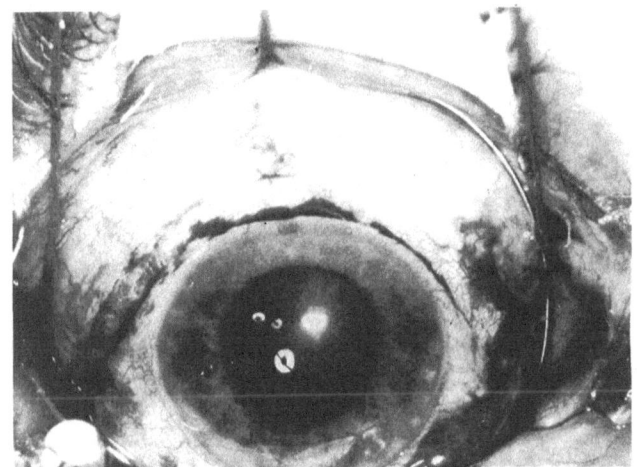

Fig. 12

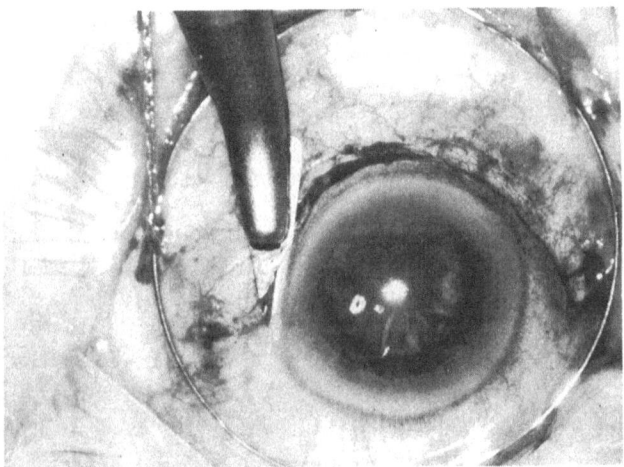

Fig. 13

are at 3 and 9 o'clock. The fornix based flap is situated at the 12 o'clock area.

This procedure of the combined limbal based and fornix based flap combines the advantages of both techniques and eliminates their disadvantages.

This section has been designed for the purpose of lensimplantation in particular, but can be used in conventional cataract surgery as well.

One particular advantage is the fact that the 12 o'clock area is almost devoid of a conjunctival flap, which now cannot interfere with lens implantation manoevres.

LAMELLAR UNDERMINING OF THE LIMBAL
BASED PART OF THE CONJUNCTIVAL SECTION.
('Meridionalisation' of the 3 and 9 o'clock areas.) Fig. 13.

The conjunctival insertion of the 12 o'clock area extends further onto the cornea than at 3 and 9 o'clock. It is of considerable help in lens implantation to create artificially the same anatomical arrangement at 3 and 9 o'clock, by surgically imitating the natural 12 o'clock anatomy of the conjunctival insertion.

This is performed by the author's lamellar intracorneal undermining procedure. A special knife has been constructed for this technique, with the correct size and inclination. This knife further has an unusual sharpness, due to a new technique in knife manufacturing. (See: The theory and practice of tissue sectioning, A new system for surgical knives. In preparation).

By 'shaving' the conjunctiva away from the limbal area a thin lamellar 'shelf' is made. The depth of the shelf can be judged best when the course of the tip of the knife is directly observed through the conjunctival insertion. (Fig. 13.)

THE HALF DEPTH INITIAL INCISION

With the same lamellar dissection knife a half depth incision is made perpendicular to the sclera, in the scleral area bordering the cornea. Due to the meridionalisation technique this section can be continued along the whole 180° circumference.

Any hemorrhages now occurring can be carefully cauterized, if there is no tendency to spontaneous coagulation. It is an essential part of this preparative technique that hemorrhages, in particular in the 3 and 9 o'clock areas, are produced before actually opening the anterior chamber. In lens implantation it is of considerable importance to keep the anterior chamber free from blood. Blood decreases visibility, which is essential for a correct positioning of the posterior loops. It further tends to cause temporary fibrinous deposits on the lens surface.

A technical guide to the making of the half depth incision: When using the autor's 45° knife for corneo-scleral sectioning the tip of the knife can be inserted in the scleral tissue to a depth equal to the width of the honed part of knife edge. A special knife is also avaible set to the desired incision depth.

The preplaced U suture. (Fig. 14)

A virgin silk preplaced suture is put half way between 10 and 11 and half way between 1 and 2 o'clock. The first stitch is placed corneo-sclerally and the second sclero-corneally. The needle is left in place bridging the half depth section. Virgin silk in lens implantation should only be used as a temporary suture. This material is insufficiently inert and perlon or steel sutures are much more preferable.

The excellent mechanical properties of virgin silk however, makes its continued use as a preliminary suture advisable.

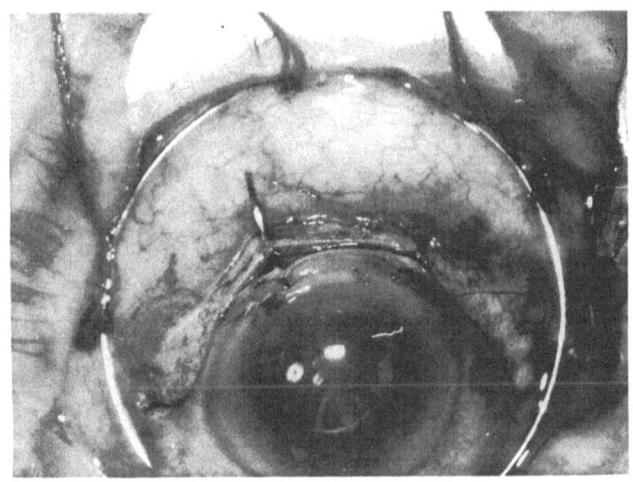

Fig. 14

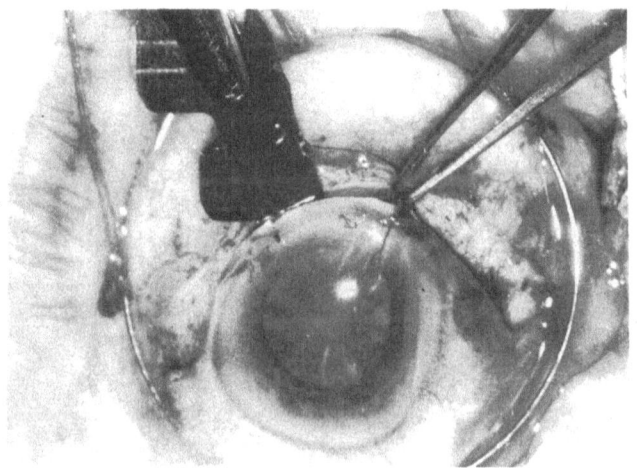

Fig. 15

Completing the corneal section.

With the author's special knife the section is carried through into the anterior chamber between the virgin silk sutures. A somewhat slanting position
of the knife edge is chosen, so as to terminate the scleral section in corneal
tissue.(Fig. 15.) While making the section the knife is directed against the
needle bridging the half depth section. (Fig. 16).In this way inadvertent
suture sectioning is effectively prevented. After making the 12 o'clock total
section the second virgin silk is pulled through. At this stage air may now be
injected to stop any further potential hemorrhages. The section is now
enlarged with Castroviejo's corneal scissors. Care should be taken not to use
a miniature type of corneal CASTROVIEJO scissors (TROUTMAN-
CASTROVIEJO) as their internal branch is not sufficiently bulky to make

53

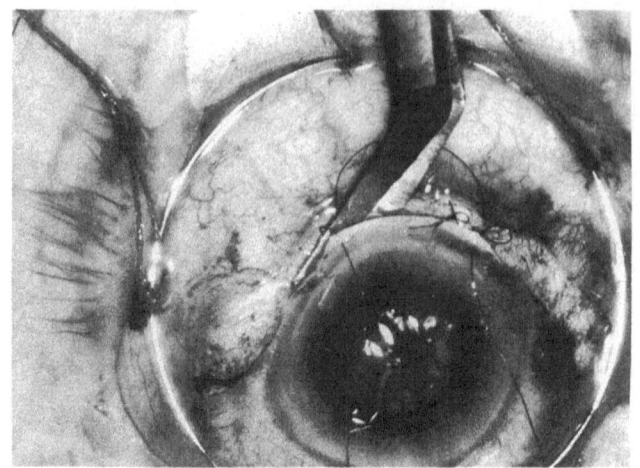

Fig. 16

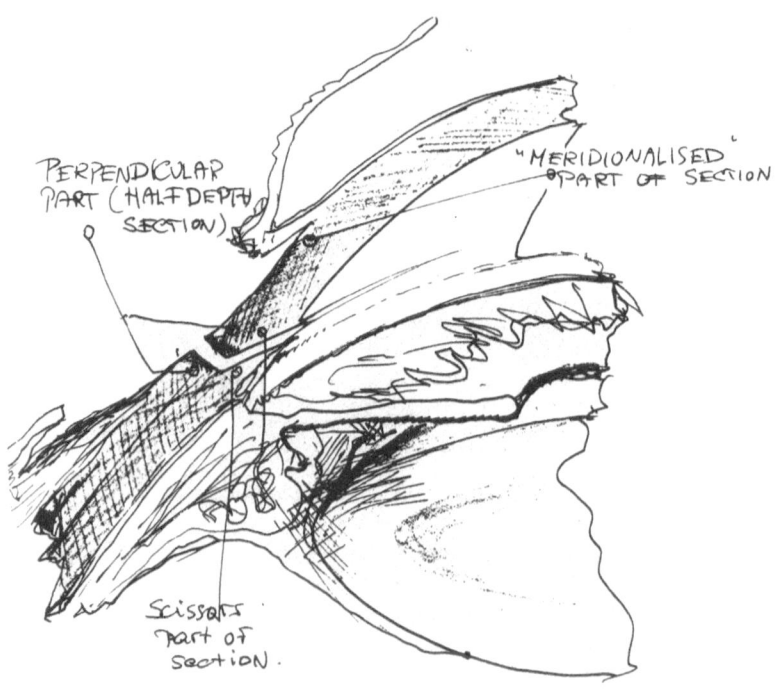

PERPENDICULAR
PART (HALFDEPTH
SECTION)

"MERIDIONALISED"
PART OF SECTION

Scissors
part of
section.

Fig. 17

the iris to slide out of the way automatically. The two step incision results
in an anatomical configuration of the wound as shown in Fig. 17.

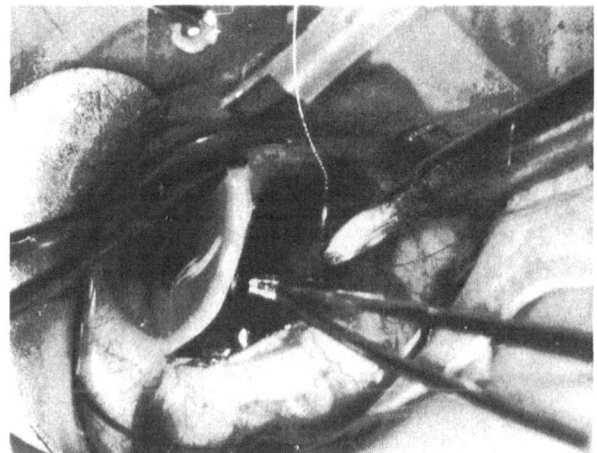

Fig. 18A

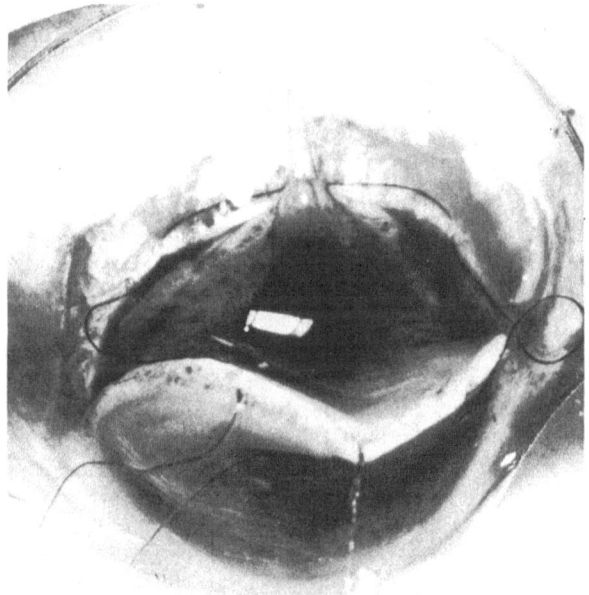

Fig. 18B

The author's procedure for advoiding inadvertent sectioning of the
virgin silk 'bridge' sutures. (Fig. 18)

It is common surgical usage to pull away the sutures bridging the half depth
section. By leaving the sutures forming a short bridge over the section one
may slip the external branch of the scissors under it. If the suture is kept
taut any chance of inadvertent suture cutting is eliminated. This technique
of 'close-in fighting' is higly recommended here. In order to facilitate the
introduction of the external length of the scissors under the suture bridge

55

the scissors have been slightly modified by the author. (The external branch has been bevelled and sharpened).

The total length of the corneal scleral section for lens implantation of the iris medallion lens should be nearly 180°.

Any effort to reduce the size of this section is useless and illadvised. It is not the purpose of the surgical technique described here to facilitate lens-extraction, but lens implantation. This dictates a large section so as to ensure the least possible damage to the corneal endothelium during implant-ation manoeuvres. As a larger section poses particular problems in wound closure a special procedure for hermetic wound closure has been designed by the author. (steel sutures, combined with the author's running stitch, see there.)

THE PLACING OF THE IRIS STITCH.

Perlon sutures for the iris stitch. Perlon sutures ŏr 30 Mu stainless steel may be used. Each suture has it specific surgical technique, which must be des-cribed seperately.

THE PERLON IRIS STITCH FOR FIXATION OF
THE IRIS MEDALLION LENS.

A special suture is provided for the purpose with a 6 mm. atraumatic needle. The Perlon suture is first passed through the episcleral tissue and knotted.
1. The first function of this step is to clean the suture of foreign bodies. The second function is to anchor it.
2. The assistant should lift the cornea.
3. The surgeon grasps the edge of the pupil at 12 o'clock and lifts it deliberately away from the lens.
4. The 6 mm. needle is passed through the iris stroma and around the sphincter muscle. A 3 mm. bite should be taken. (To judge this length one may make estimate from the length of the needle.) The tip of the needle is presented in the pupil. (Fig. 18A shows this phase). Only then the needle is passed backwards of the iris again and pushed through the iris stroma for-wards.
5. The tip of the needle is grasped with the forceps.
6. The needleholder is used to massage the iris gently over the needle until sufficient length of the tip becomes visible to permit its grasping with the needle holder. Do not attempt to grasp the tip immediately with the needle holder as iris stroma may be grasped with it.
7. Pull some 10 cm. of suture through the iris and do not remove the needle.

THE IRIS STITCH PERFORMED WITH A 30Mu
STAINLESS STEEL SUTURE.

1. The suture is passed through the sclera as described with the Perlon suturing technique. Other phases are the same up to point 6. The steel suture should be bent slightly at its point of entry in the sclera. (This replaces the knot on the Perlon stitch.)

2. The steel suture should be cut at ± 1 cm. from its point of emergence from the anterior chamber. (The Perlon stitch is left much longer) After putting in the fixation iris stitch of Perlon or steel one may now decide whether extra- or intracapsular extraction will be used.

The decision and the indication for taking the one technique or the other will be discussed under: 'extra- versus intracapsular extraction:' Indications technique and complications (in preparation)

This paper deals with routine intracapsular surgery only.

IRIS RETRACTION PROCEDURES.

As an iris stitch has been placed, this very same stitch may be used to retract the iris for kryoextraction. (Fig. 18B). In case of a steel suture this manoeuvre is particularly effective due to the relative stiffness of the steel suture.

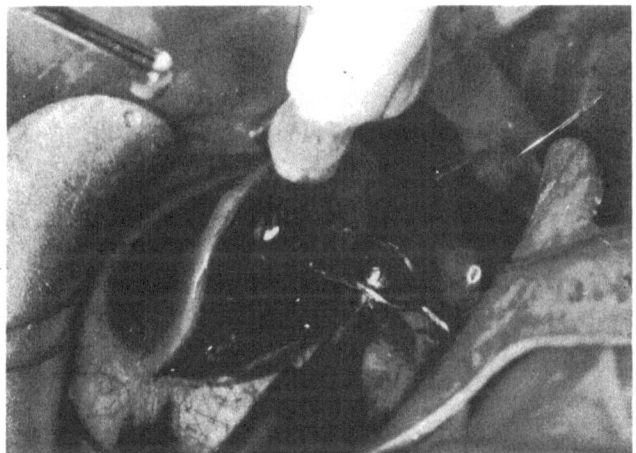

Fig. 19

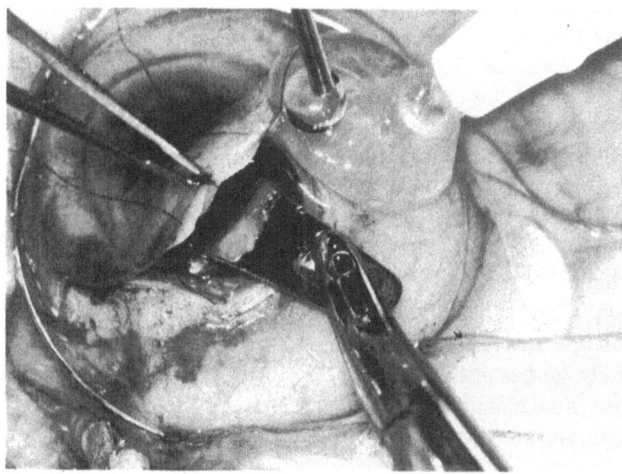

Fig. 20

As an alternative procedure one may either use the author's adjustable retractor (Fig. 20) or the author's miniature iris retractor (Fig. 19). This is particularly useful when stitch retraction fails to produce sufficient space for the extractor.

The miniature retractor (The iris 'beatle') has its inbuilt grasping hooks to hold itself to the sclera (Fig. 19). This retractor will lift itself away from the iris spontaneously after completion of lensextraction. In our experience this retractor is less traumatic than handheld types of iris retractors. One such retractor, the authors adjustable iris retractor, is shown in Fig. 20.

After succesful kryoextraction the moment of truth has arrived to decide whether a lens can be implanted. For beginners in this field it is strongly recommended only to perform lens implantation when there is no bulging of the vitreous surface.

TECHNIQUE OF IMPLANTATION OF THE IRIS MEDALLION LENS.

With Perlon suture. The lens is removed from its sterilizing container and placed in the neutralizing container before starting surgery. After removing it from the neutralizing container it should be kept in a bowl of balanced salt solution. The lens is grasped at the haptic edge with a simple needle holder. For the right eye it grasped at the right, for the left eye it grasped at the left. *Inspection should now follow of the lens under the microscope for foreign body contamination, and to ascertain that the lens is in optimal condition. Observe the position of the loops in particular.*

The lens has electrostatic properties and may attract foreign bodies, when transported through the air. It further tends to collect foreign bodies from the saline solutions on the surgical table. First the needle of the Perlon stitch is now passed through the left hole in the iris medallion lens, from behind forwards and than passed from front to back through the right hole. The suture should carefully be kept stretched by the assistant to prevent snaring around the posterior loops while inserting the lens in the pupil. This is an essential part of the procedure.

With the steel suture these tricky parts of the Perlon procedure can be omitted. For the special lens for steel suture see: lens design. The lens is than placed in the pupil, first beginning with an open sky manoeuvre, but finishing the insertion by observing the lens through the cornea. Some pressure towards the vitreous body must be exerted, and great care should be taken not to rub the lens against the corneal endothelium.

Note: The lens is placed in the pupil with a rotational movement not unlike the throwing of a 'Frisbee'. Note further that the backward stroke must be made first and that the posterior loop nearest to the free hand of the surgeon is placed second. It may be necessary to perform some forceps traction on the iris root to dilate the pupil mechanically. If the required backhand stroke has not been made the surgeon finds himself unable to perform this essential manual aid, (unless he can work 'crosshanded').

Pilocarpin (intraocular pilocarpin 'Meram') or acetylcholine is now used to constrict the pupil. Pilocarpine is preferred, as this is a pharmacologically stable solution.

It is essential that the iris stitch is not tightened too much. The stitch serves only as a prevention against lens luxation and should only maintain the lens near the upper pupillary border. To close the suture, the knotted end attached to the sclera is cut free. (*Do not forget!*) A single knot is now made and repeated three times. While tying the knot it will be noticed that the free ends of the knot will bury themselves spontaneously under the haptic rim of the lens. The knotting of the sutures can be performed with the corneo-scleral wound in apposition. It is not necessary to use an open sky technique. The absence of a conjunctival flap at 12 o'clock greatly facilitates this part of the operation.

The free ends emerging from under the lens are now cut flush with the lens edge. This prevents touch of the corneal endothelium effectively.

IRIDECTOMY

It is only at this point of the operation that an iridectomy must be made. The making of an iridectomy prior to lens extraction is strongly dissuaded.

It may cause local vitreous problems in the iridectomy and the iridectomy may interfere with free movements of the posterior loops of the lens during insertion. Care should be taken that the iridectomy is not made too periferal and that it opens the space between the lens edge and the perifery effectively. A single iridectomy is sufficient. Make sure the pigment layer is also opened!

THE STEEL IRIS SUTURE:

The steel suture is mechanically very different from the Perlon stitch, because it is highly unelastic.

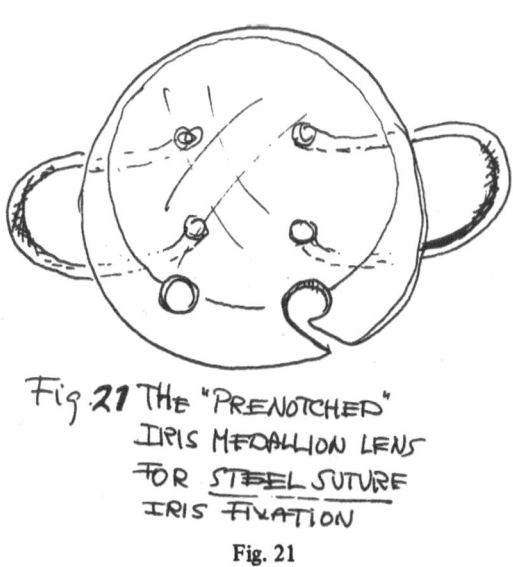

Fig. 21 THE "PRENOTCHED" IRIS MEDALLION LENS FOR STEEL SUTURE IRIS FIXATION

Fig. 21

The steel suture is placed in exactly the same manner as the Perlon stitch. However, it is cut short at 1 cm. from its point of emergence from the corneal scleral wound. Its opposite end is not fastened to the sclera with a knot, but may be temporarily hooked to subconjunctival tissue.

The steel suture is particularly suited to serve as an iris retractor. For its use in iris medallion lens fixation the lens must be modified slightly. One notch must be cut in the side of the haptic rim. The notch is connected with the right hole. (see Fig. 21) 'Prenotched' lenses are also avaible on request.

TECHNIQUE FOR CLOSING THE STEEL IRIS SUTURE (IRIS STAPLING TECHNIQUE)

The assistant lifts the cornea and grasps the right end of the steel suture to give some counter traction if necessary. The surgeon grasps the lens at the haptic edge and passes the free end of the suture through the left hole. The lens is implanted. The grasp of the lens is than shifted, to include the end of the suture in the grasp. The right end of the suture is, grasped with a second needle holder and passed through the right slotted hole. The two free ends of the staple suture are stretched and cut short. Care must be taken to push the free ends against the anterior surface of the lens after cutting.

In practice this procedure proved simpler than the author's original Perlon iris medallion lens stitch.

It presupposes however a considerable amount of practice with steel sutures and the risks involved in this steel stapling technique seem somewhat higher than with the Perlon stitch. In particular the stiffness of the steel stitch may cause problems. This stapling technique is based on the physical behaviour of steel which bends extremely easily. The final 'suture' is a straight 'pin', with a slightly bayonetted shape in the holes (Fig. 22).

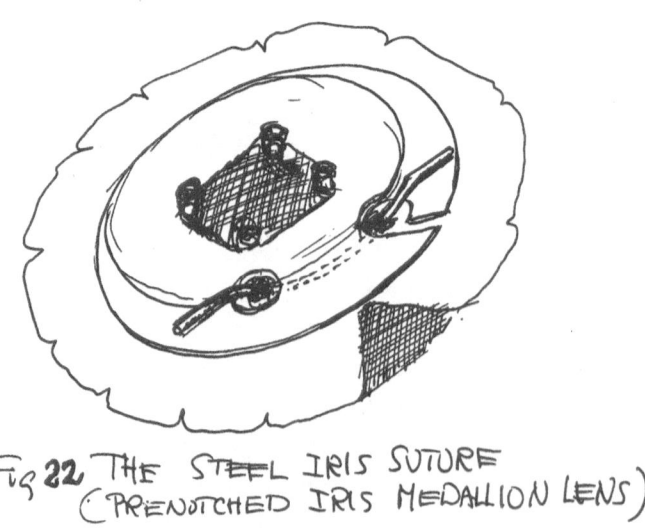

Fig 22 THE STEEL IRIS SUTURE
(PRENOTCHED IRIS MEDALLION LENS)

Fig. 22

60

The virgin silk U suture is separated in the middle and the two separate sutures thus produced are knotted.

No effort should be made to cut the sutures short as they will be removed at a later stage. At this stage an air injection must be performed to protect the cornea from being rubbed against the lens during the suturing.

The technique of air injection is deceptively simple but is in fact a dangerous phase of the operation as air may slip behind the lens or through the iridectomy. To prevent this Binkhorst manoeuvre is highly effective. At the moment of air injection the assistant should depress the center of the cornea slightly. This results in a doughnut shaped form of the air bubble, which is the aerodynamically favourable shape to prevent air from slipping behind the lens. Previous lack of knowledge of this particular step of the operation has already caused several times the complication of air entering the posterior chamber.

Air in the posterior chamber may be difficult to remove and may cause airbloc (see: Pitfalls and complications of artificial lens surgery).

STEEL SUTURES FOR CORNEO-SCLERAL WOUND CLOSURE

The author has used 30 Mu steel suture systematically for corneo-scleral wound suturing over a period of 3 years. He has found that the advantages over conventional suturing materials are considerable. Steel suturing has become a standard procedure for wound closure in any type of lens implantation.

Some advantages of 30 Mu stainless steel sutures:
1. The material is excessively strong (± 10 x Perlon)
2. The knot of a steel suture, if made according to the author's technique is extremely strong.
3. Steel is a totally inert material, which can also be used intra-ocularly.
4. The material is easy to handle.
5. It can be applied without free suture ends protruding from the knot.
6. It is easy to sterilize.

TECHNIQUE FOR PLACING A 30 Mu. STAINLESS STEEL SUTURE

The needle is passed through the corneo-scleral section with a short bite. A double throw is now made and the knot is tightened with considerable traction. Care must be taken to shift the position of the hands while tightening the knot, otherwise the steel suture may kink. However, if a kink is present simple bilateral traction on the suture will undo this kink. If too large a bite has been taken this may be corrected by making three throws. The free ends of the knot must now be cut flush with the surface. This hides the cut below the smooth loops formed by the double throws.

For details of steel suturing technique, see Fig. 23A, B, C.

Fig. 23A: Two needleholder techniques for loop formation.

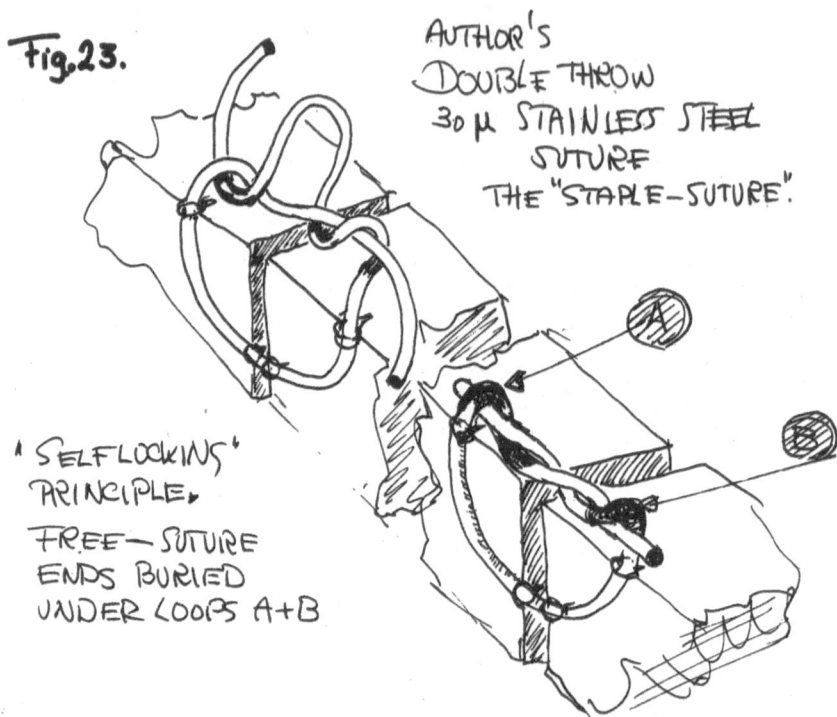

Fig.23.

AUTHOR'S
DOUBLE THROW
30 μ STAINLESS STEEL
SUTURE
THE "STAPLE—SUTURE"

'SELFLOCKING'
PRINCIPLE.

FREE—SUTURE
ENDS BURIED
UNDER LOOPS A+B

Fig. 23

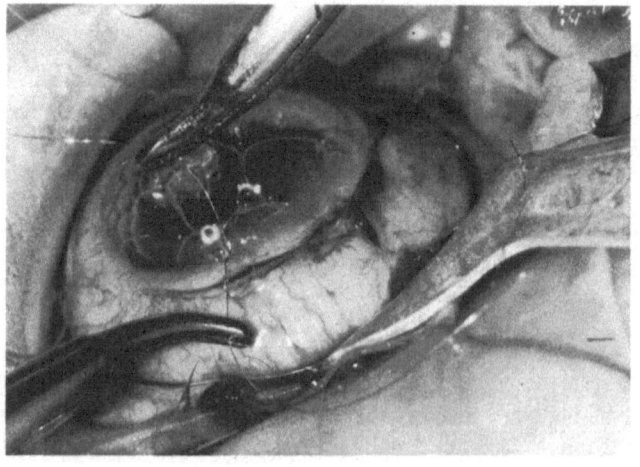

Fig. 23A

Fig. 23B: Fully closed knot.

Fig. 23C: Technique for cutting free suture ends flush with the scleral surface.

To cut the sutures without leaving protruding ends, (which would create a 'barbed wire' effect) the scissors are slipped along the suture against the knot and while exerting some downward pressure the suture is cut. It may

62

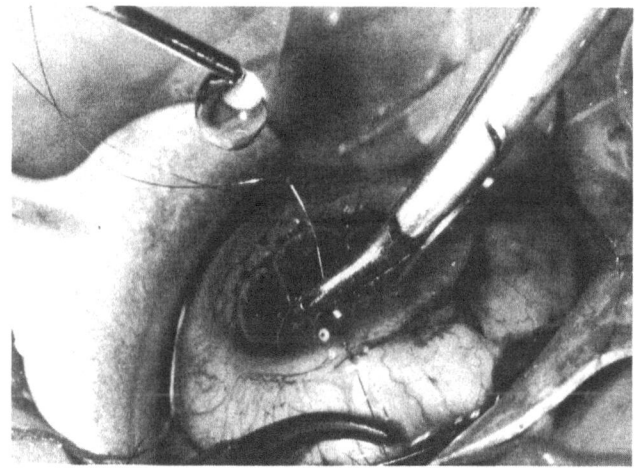

Fig. 23B

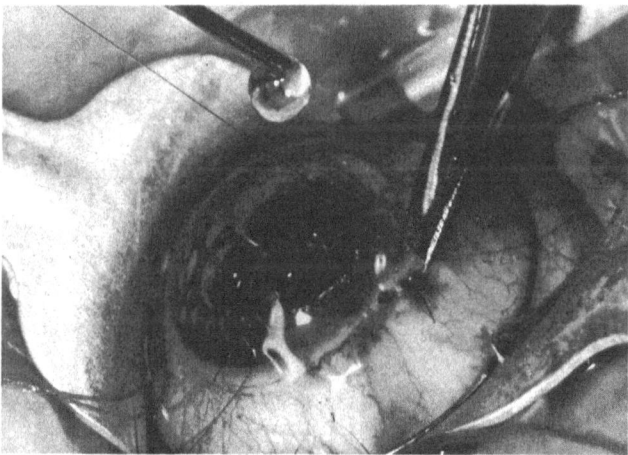

Fig. 23C

be useful to perform this act under a microscope. Fig. 24 shows some finished steel corneo-scleral sutures

THE NUMBER OF STEEL STITCHES

A test for ascertaining whether sufficient stitches have been placed

When some 8 stitches have been placed one should put traction on the conjunctiva between the sutures and observe the behaviour of the wound edges. If some gaping still occurs an intermediate stitch must be placed. Generally some 10 to 15 stitches are required for hermetic wound closure.

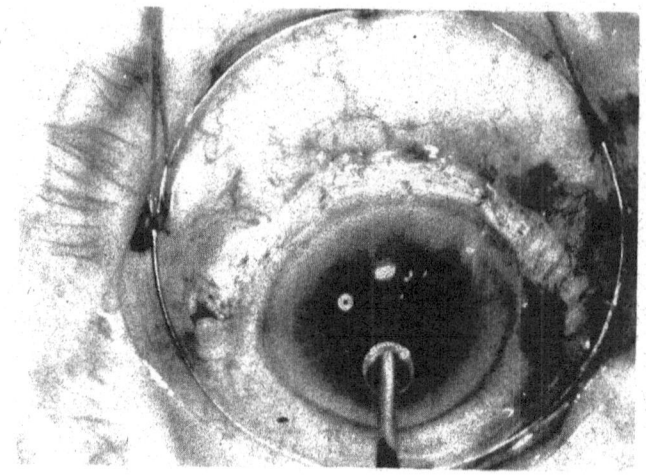

Fig. 24

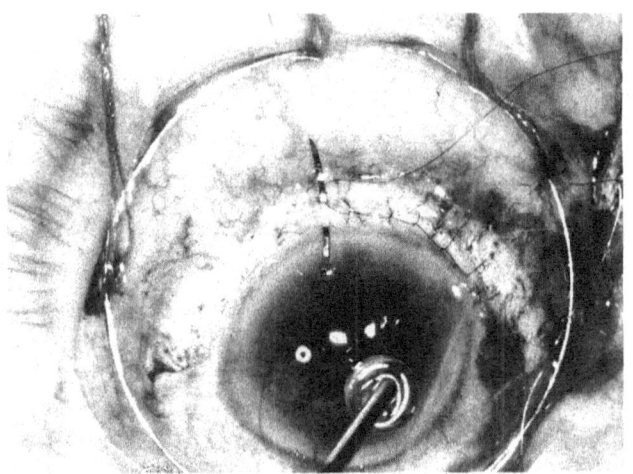

Fig. 25

THE ADDITIONAL PERLON STITCH

(The author's knotted running stitch)

Previous to the steel sutures the author has been using the 'knotted running stitch'. The stitch is still used as an additional wound closure in conjunction with the steel sutures.

THE TECHNIQUE OF THE KNOTTED RUNNING STITCH

In the left end of the wound (for a right handed surgeon) an initial stitch is made and knotted. The needle is than passed through the wound edges, but left in place. (Fig. 25).

The suture is now passed between the tip and the end of the needle, from left to right and passed backwards under the needle tip.

If the needle is now pulled out a half knot will be formed. The suture is finally pulled to the left first and than tightened by pulling it to the right. For the next stitch the sequence is repeated.

The knotted running stitch has first been described during a meeting of the French Society in 1964

The advantages of this suturing technique are that each stitch has its own belaying point. It is also possible to use the technique without half knots. The essence of the procedure however is lost therewith. A copy of this technique by MAUMENEE uses incorrect half knots, which tend to slip.

Note: If during wound closure air should escape it must be replaced immediately.

TECHNIQUE FOR EXCHANGING AIR FOR SALINE

At the end of suturing the air must be removed quantitatively. This is done by bringing a fine air canula deep in the anterior chamber, in contact with the center of the artificial lens. The lens is somewhat depressed while air is removed by suction; saline should now be injected at the same time, to prevent arterior chamber collapse.

SALINE INJECTION

Saline can now be injected but care should be taken not to raise the pressure too much. Normal manual syringe pressure is already far above physiological values. Wound closure with steel, in particular when combined with the running stitch is so effective that no leakage can occur, which might balance overpressure.

A further technical detail is the injection at various places between the sutures, to loosen up any temporary synechial formations in the chamber angle.

INSPECTION OF THE ANTERIOR CHAMBER
WITH THE MICROSCOPE

If the microscope has not been used during the whole procedure one must now perform inspection with the microscope, to check if any foreign bodies have been introduced. Also the position of the lens and of the iris suture must be checked. It is useful to finish the intraocular part of the operation by pushing the lens downwards during the saline injection, to give it an optimal centration.

The removal of the Flieringa ring. By cutting the stitches with a Gilette blade the ring can be easily removed. Scissors should not be used to cut these sutures as short ends of suture will be left in the sclera. The best way to cut the suture is to slide the Gilette blade over the ring until it touches the knot. The knot should be kept stretched when cutting it by exerting traction on the suture.

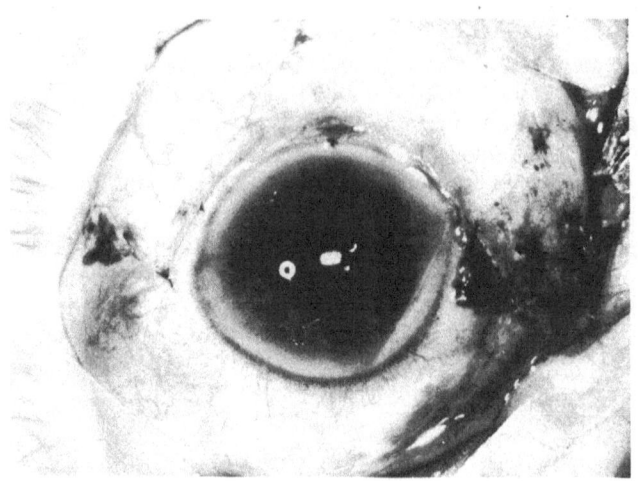

Fig. 26

CLOSURE OF THE CONJUNCTIVA (Fig. 26)

Several interrupted virgin silk sutures can be used to close the 'straight' conjunctival wound. Note, that some subconjunctival wound tissue contraction always occurs. This subconjunctival tissue contraction can be released grasping the conjunctival flap and mobilizing it by traction.

POSTOPERATIVE CARE

If in doubt, a prophylactic antibiotic treatment should be given. This is not a standard part of the procedure however. A local steroid and an antibiotic are instilled 6 x daily.

This is diminished after a week to 3 x daily. Most cases will be without topical medication after 4 weeks.

No miotics or mydriatics should be used with the iris medallion lens. The natural movement of the pupil is effective to prevent too much synechial formation. Some synechial formation at the upper pupillary border is frequent and desirable however. In a routine case the postoperative reaction is little more than in a standard case of cataract extraction without lens implantation. The cornea however is usually more cloudy for several days.

This is due to contact of the intraocular lens with the endothelium during surgery.

If it has been possible to insert a lens without any endothelial contact one will see a completely clear cornea the next day.

For early and late postoperative complications see: Pitfalls and complications of artificial lens surgery. (in preparation)

SUMMARY

A description of the surgical technique for implantation of the 'iris medallion lens'.

66

REFERENCE

BINKHORST, C.D.: The iridocapsular (two-loop) lens and the iris-clip (four-loop) lens in pseudophakia. Transactions American Academy of Ophthalmology and Otolaryngology, sept.-okt. 1973.

Author's address:
J.G.F. Worst
Dept. of Ophthalmology
Refaja Hospital
Stadskanaal
The Netherlands

ARTIFICIAL LENSDESIGN

J.G.F. WORST

(Haren, Gr.)

INTRODUCTION

Since the first practical realization of an artificial lens by HAROLD RIDLEY a large number of modifications of intraocular lenses have appeared. These lenses differ in basic design and in their methods of support by the intraocular structures. It seemed of interest to review and consider the merits and demerits of some of the existing types of lenses and to describe a number of variations which have been used succesfully, in order to determine which type of lens design is the optimal solution for a given situation. It will be evident that no single type of lens can be considered the ultimate solution for artificial lens surgery.

RIDLEY'S POSTERIOR CHAMBER LENS

Fig. 1.

All intraocular artificial lenswork starts with the epochal discovery of RIDLEY that it was possible to insert an artificial lens made of methylmethacrylate inside the eye.

A number of late complications did manifest themselves but, contrary to the general belief these complications were not of a biochemical nature in the first place, but mainly due to the *physical* presence of the Ridley lens. Ridley's lens was too heavy to be supported permanently by the posterior capsule alone.

The clinical sequence, which was obviously often observed, of a progressive deterioration of the eye overshadowed the fact that a number of Ridley lenses were inserted succesfully and remained without problems and good function for many years. The attention shou'¹ have been directed towards the succesful cases to explain this succes instead of turning to the insuccesful cases to explain the failures.

If this had been done in the first place the story of artificial lenses would have been a positive one instead of what it has become now: A long history of failures to insert artificial lenses after cataract surgery, until BINKHORST succeeded to find a practical solution.

The basic idea of RIDLEY has been so sound and so succesful that it is deplorable that only the fact that his lens was still too large and therefore too heavy decreased the succes rate in an inacceptable manner.

Later in time certain developments have returned to Ridley's original posterior capsule fixation (BINKHORST).

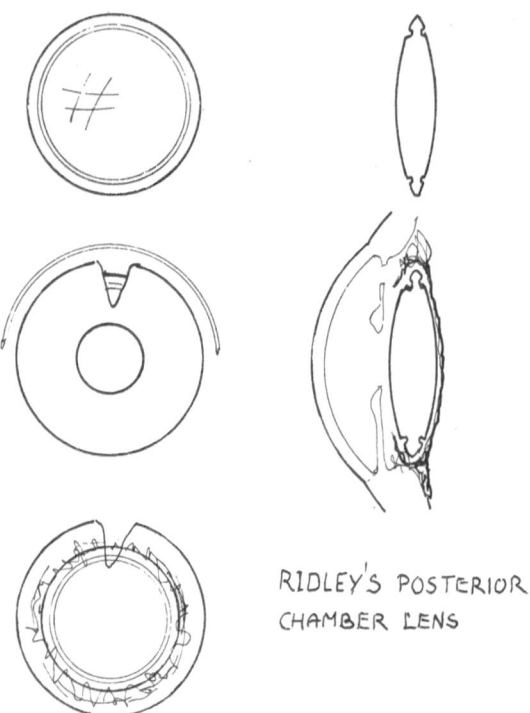

RIDLEY'S POSTERIOR CHAMBER LENS

Fig. 1

Fig. 1 shows Ridley's posterior chamber lens with its special rim for better fixation with a special grasping forceps.

This rim has been another cause of late failures as the first lenses tended to retain foreign material. Ridley's lens could only be slipped in after a succesful extracapsular extraction. The basic idea of RIDLEY to use the posterior capsule for fixation and the posterior chamber for placing the optical part of the lens has been the example for the author to insert the optical part of Binkhorst's lenses behind the pupil by inverting this lens.

The author's iris medallion has also been inserted in an inverted manner to bring the whole lens in the posterior chamber. Inverted lenses have been implanted in intra- and extracapsular cases succesfully. The reason for inverting a lens however has not been to change the mode of fixation but to reduce the power of the lens for optical reasons only. A lens which has been designed for posterior chamber placement is the inverted 'scarabee' iris medallion lens (Fig. 22, see there).

(Fig. 2).

The lens uses the posterior capsule as a support, together with some periferal capsular remains (Soemmering's ring). The optical part of Binkhorst iridocapsular lens is situated in front of the iris. In view of the highly succesful method of BINKHORST, using extracapsular technique and capsule fixation it seemed possible to reconsider implantation of an artificial lens according

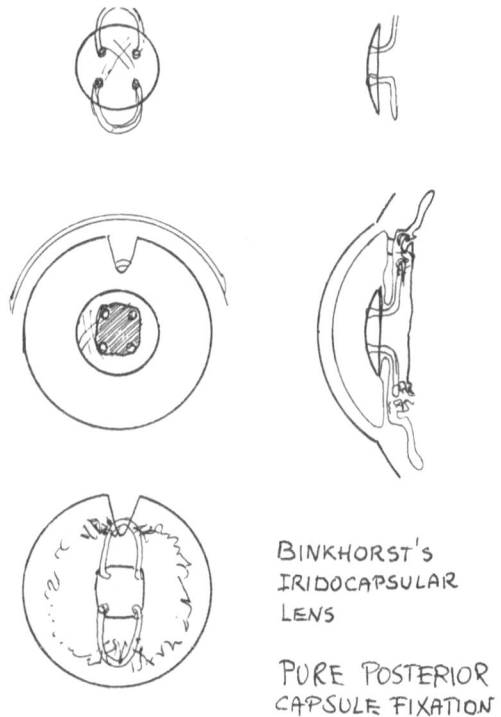

BINKHORST'S
IRIDOCAPSULAR
LENS

PURE POSTERIOR
CAPSULE FIXATION

Fig. 2

to RIDLEY. Ridley's lens had to be redesigned in order to remove its only defect: Too much weight.

REDUCED SIZE AND WEIGHT POSTERIOR CHAMBER LENS (PRINCIPLE DESIGN)

(Fig. 3).

Fig. 3 shows the principle design of a modified Ridley lens. The optical part has been reduced to the minimum necessary and the haptic part has been cut away leaving only a periferal supporting ring. The notch at the 12 o'clock position of this lens has been added to facilitate insertion through a relatively narrow pupil. In order to make use of this notch the lens should

71

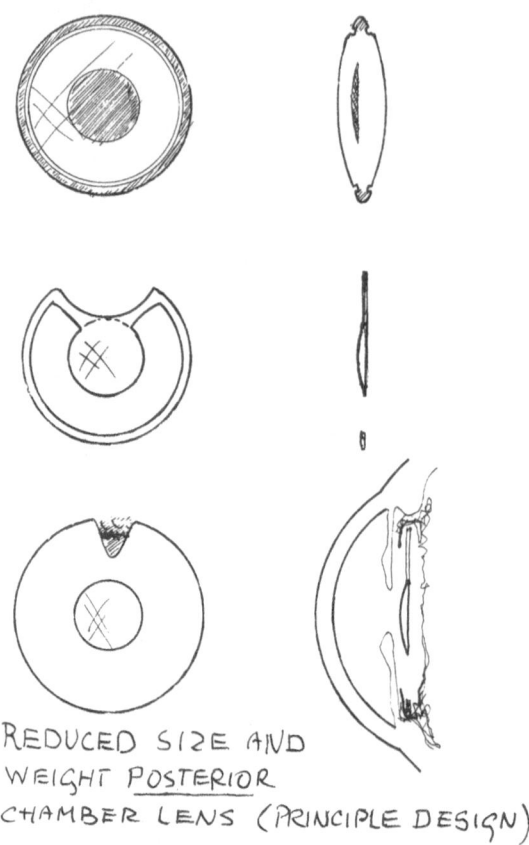

REDUCED SIZE AND
WEIGHT POSTERIOR
CHAMBER LENS (PRINCIPLE DESIGN)

Fig. 3

be rotated during insertion. Lenses of this type have been made but have not been implanted by the author as yet.

The reason to refrain from using this design is the fact that other lens-designs are highly succesful wherefore further development in lensdesign seems relatively pointless. An obvious disadvantage of the principle design of Fig. 3 is the fact that a large incision is required for this type of lens. It is conceiveable however that this principle design can be used for a lens which can be inserted through a small opening. Some research along this line is in progress at the moment. In the author's opinion the original Ridley principle, supported by the experience with Binkhorst's iridocapsular fixation of his anterior chamber lens may lead to a further development of the original Ridley lens. In the cases in which the author has implanted lenses of various designs, including his own iris medallion lens he has noticed a reduction of photophobia in the cases which have received the lens in the posterior chamber. This is probably due to the fact that the pupil can now constrict to its minimal size required for daylight conditions. All anterior chamber lenses with posterior chamber support cause some sort of pupil stop which under unfavourable lighting conditions, results in photophobia.

Fig. 4.

Fig. 4 shows a modified model of Fig. 3 with titanium posterior loops. In the designing of new anterior chamber lenses the possibility of full dilatation and full pupil constriction must always be considered. In an effort to

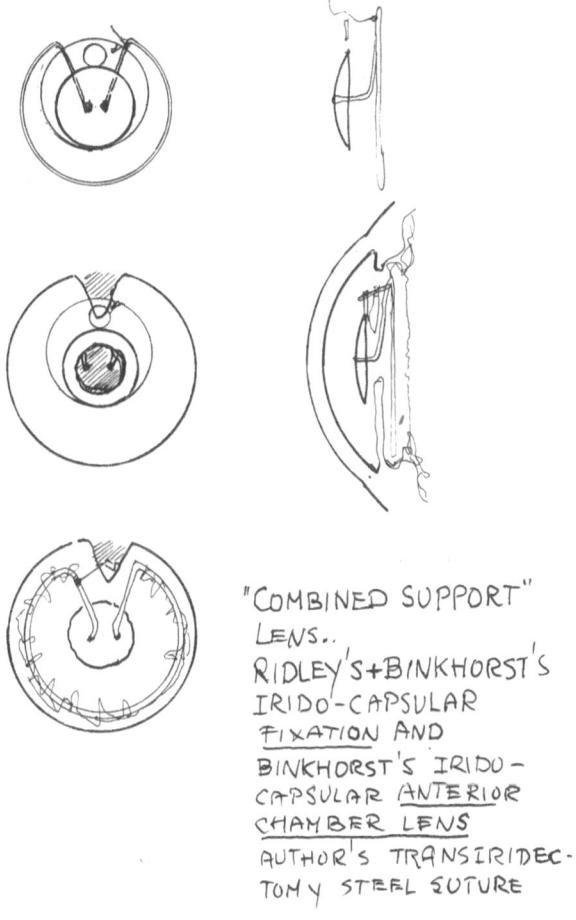

"COMBINED SUPPORT"
LENS..
RIDLEY'S+BINKHORST'S
IRIDO-CAPSULAR
FIXATION AND
BINKHORST'S IRIDO-
CAPSULAR ANTERIOR
CHAMBER LENS
AUTHOR'S TRANSIRIDEC-
TOMY STEEL SUTURE

Fig. 4

overcome the disadvantages of Ridley's lens a number of author's have designed the so-called anterior chamber lenses. (STRAMPELLI).

Fig. 5.

A host of different types of anterior chamber lenses followed Strampelli's modification. All these lenses used the chamber angle as anatomical support. These lenses are of historical interest only. It is remarkable how many of these lenses in a short period of time have been implanted with usually a lack of clinical follow-up which would have rapidly demonstrated the basic fallacy of this procedure: Internal damage to the endothelium leading to corneal dystrophy. It is STRAMPELLI himself who was among the first to realize the basic error in the design of all chamber angle supported lenses.

STRAMPELLI has repeatedly warned against this principle. Nevertheless too many authors have continued to modify the anterior angle supported lenses. A rough estimate of the number of cases which have received these lenses has yielded a figure of ± 3000 - 3500. This figure cannot be found in ophthalmic surgical literature as many of the failures with anterior chamber lenses have not been reported. An exception must be made for a communication by JOAQUIN BARRAQUER who has implanted 400 lenses of his own design (Fig. 5, J) and has observed in the course of some 10 years, more than 50% functional or anatomical loss in this series. This has been an incentive for BARRAQUER to abandon all artificial lens work, on the assumption that any artificial lens would finally produce the same extremely high rate of late complications (in particular: corneal dystrophy.)

While these lenses were still being used elsewhere, BINKHORSTs, in Holland has designed the pupil supported lens which showed none of the higher rate of complications of the anterior chamber angle lenses. This breakthrough in artificial lens work has remained relatively unnoticed for a long period. One reason for this is the preconceived idea that also this system would fail in the long run. Some 15 years of experience with a total number of about 4500 cases in Holland are proof to the contrary. For historical interest we have made a principle design of some anterior chamber artificial lenses. (Fig. 5.)

The basic idea is Strampelli's lens, A (1950).

B. is Strampelli's lens with backward curved haptic parts.

C. is a lens proposed by APPOLLONIO.

D. Barron's lens (1953).

E. F.G. are designs by BIETTI.

H. is Chreck's lens.

I. Dannheim's lens.

J. is Barraquer's modification of Dannheim's lens.

K. is Lieb-Dupont-Guerry-Gerraets lens.

L. is Strampelli's trans-scleral external fixation lens.

M. and N. Boberg-Ans modifications.

O. and P. are Choyce's modifications of the original Strampelli lens.

This series is incomplete and only serves to show the wide variety on the basic theme of chamber angle supported lenses.

In fact the modifications are only apparant and all types are based on the original Strampelli concept.

Fig. 6.

Fig. 6 shows the basic design of a Strampelli lens.

Not all anterior chamber lenses have been categorically abandoned. It is CHOYCE who has continued the use of a Strampelli lens, modified by himself. The question has been raised why in Choyce's series the number of dystrophies is much lower than in Strampelli's series.

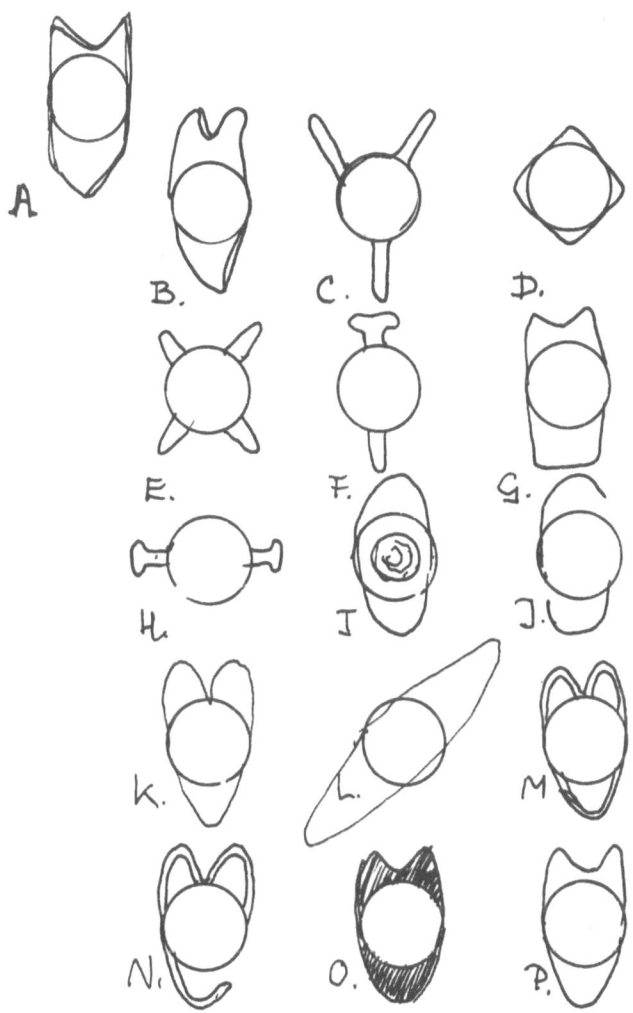

A.

B.

C.

D.

E.

F.

G.

H.

J.

J.

K.

L.

M.

N.

O.

P.

Fig. 5

Fig. 7.

Fig. 7 is giving a possible explanation.

The diameter of Choyce's lens is carefully chosen to be equal to or somewhat larger than the largest diameter of the anterior chamber measured at the iris root. In this manner the feet of the Choyce anterior chamber implant do not touch the endothelium and will therefore not produce an endothelial dystrophy.

Fig. 8.

Fig. 8 shows Strampelli's transscleral fixation principle.

This is another example of a type of fixation which uses the chamber angle

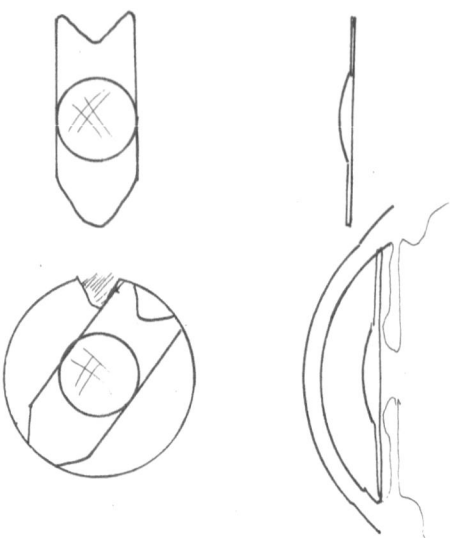

STRAMPELLI'S CHAMBER
ANGLE SUPPORTED ARTIFICIAL
LENS. (REJECTED BY
ITS AUTHOR).

Fig. 6

as a point of support without producing corneal dystrophy. Strampelli's lens has been a failure, but Strampelli's system for transscleral fixation has proven a very useful procedure for lensfixation in extremely difficult cases when destruction of the iris border or other traumatic conditions prevent proper fixation on the iris itself.

Fig. 9.

Fig. 9 This shows Epstein's 'Maltese Cross' lens.

This four flanged lens is inserted in the pupil, but the iris is 'woven' around the four haptic flanges. EPSTEIN has abandoned this system because of formation of retro-lental membranes, (Thickening of the vitreous surface?), late anterior chamber hemorrhages, intractable iritis, iris atrophy and lens luxation. The reason for these irritative phenomena seems to me the incessant movement of the iris to light which keeps on rubbing both front and rear part of the iris against the four supporting flanges.

This lens violates the basic principle put forward by BINKHORST that an artificial lens should have minimal or preferable no contact with the iris surface.

76

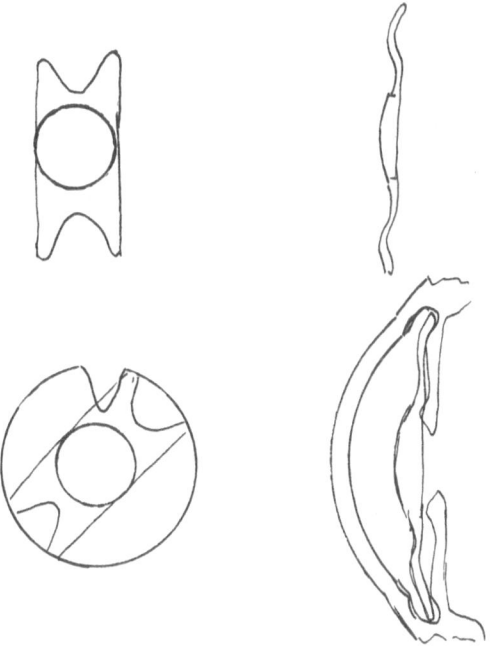

CHOYCE'S ANTERIOR CHAMBER
"ANGLE-SUPPORTED" ARTIFICIAL LENS.
CAREFUL CHOYCE OF LARGEST
POSSIBLE HAPTICS TURNS THIS LENS
INTO AN IRIS (BASE) SUPPORTED LENS.

Fig. 7

Fig. 10.

Fig. 10 shows the original Binkhorst iris clip lens.

This lens should be inserted vertically in order to prevent the anterior loops from touching the endothelium when too much iridodonesis is present. BINKHORST has added to this original technique the fixation of the anterior and posterior loops through the 12 o'clock iridectomy, by means of a suture.

This lens is giving excellent results and is widely used. The transiridectomy suture fixation effectively prevents lensluxation. In the original Binkhorst lens fixation has obtained by administration of Pilocarpin. This type of implantation and transiridectomy fixation is mainly used in intracapsular lens surgery.

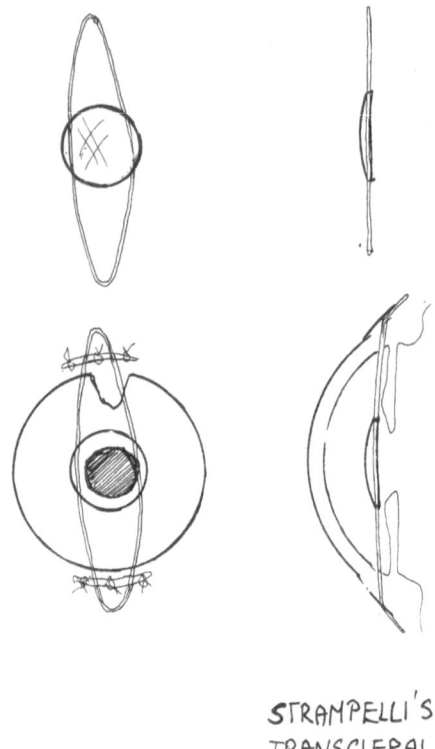

STRAMPELLI'S
TRANSCLERAL
FIXATION

Fig. 8

Fig. 11.

Several modifications of Binkhorst's lens have appeared.
2. Fedorov's crossed loop type of Binkhorst's lens.
3. Leonard's modification.
4. Fedorov's 'Sputnik' lens with 3 posterior and 3 anterior supporting elements. This lens is widely used in Russia.
5. Binkhorst's lens with black posterior loops for better visualization during the implantation.

None of these modifications are basicly different from Binkhorst's original four loop lens. The addition of an anterior or a posterior supporting element does not make a lens essentially different from the basic idea of BINKHORST.

Fig. 12.

In order to facilitate fixation, the author has introduced the use of Perlon iris sutures for fixation of artificial lenses in 1968.

Fig. 12 is showing several types of fixation of a Binkhorst lens.
1. Sutureless fixation with horizontal implantation. Fixation is obtained by

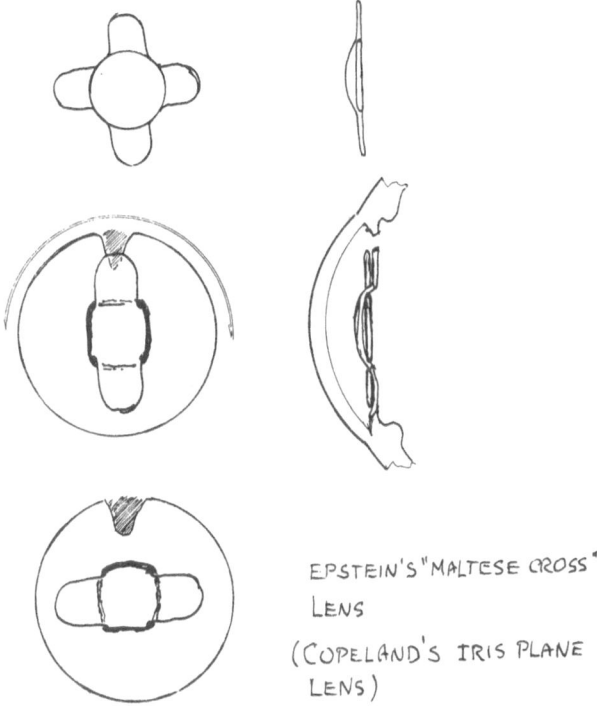

EPSTEIN'S "MALTESE CROSS" LENS
(COPELAND'S IRIS PLANE LENS)

Fig. 9

Pilocarpin administration. Note, that this position of the Binkhorst lens is incorrect. Only vertical implantation should be used.

2. Two anterior loop sutures.

3. Correct vertical implantation with Pilocarpin fixation.

4. Transstromal fixation with two sutures of the superior loop.

5. Partial closure of coloboma with iris sutures for lens fixation.

6. Closure of radial iridectomy, with inclusion of artificial lens.

7. Transstromal posterior loop fixation.

8. Inverted lensimplantation with posterior loop fixation to anterior iris surface.

9. Transiridectomy loop fixation.

10. Single loop fixation.

11. Adaptation of Binkhorst's lens to traumatic cases by means of iris sutures.

12. Shows no lensimplantation as the peaked pupil indicates vitreous loss has occurred. Vitreous loss in general is a contra-indication to lensimplantation. In particular cases however lensimplantation can be performed, after vitrectomy.

The trans-iridectomy fixation principle of Fig. 12 drawing 9, proved so useful that a special lens has been designed to facilitate transiridectomy fixation.

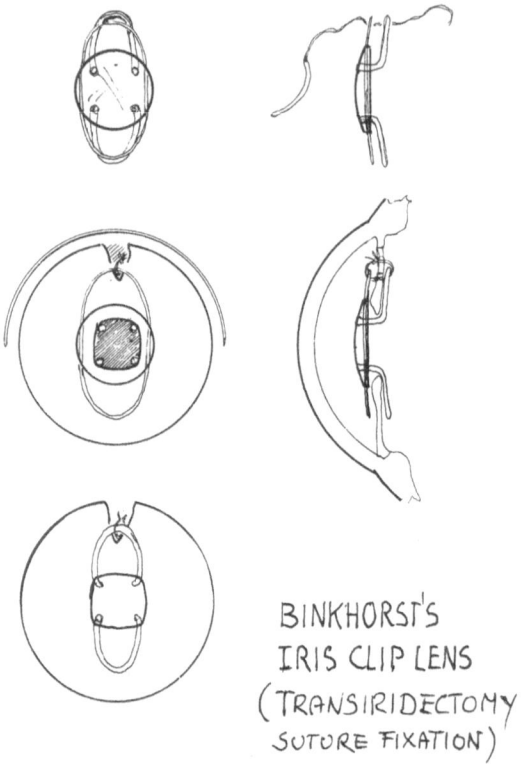

BINKHORST'S
IRIS CLIP LENS
(TRANSIRIDECTOMY
SUTURE FIXATION)

Fig. 10

Fig. 13.

Fig. 13. shows the iris medallion lens with an inbuilt transiridectomy safety clip fixation. This lens has been used in ± 150 cases and few complications have occurred. It should be noted however that the inferior loop may luxate and that the clip closure through the iridectomy must be performed most carefully. In cases where clip closure was incomplete luxations have been observed.

Fig. 14

This is the same lens as of Fig. 13, but with reduced horizontal diameters. The purpose of this lens is: insertion as a secondary procedure through a relatively narrow, preferably temporal incision. This lens is the author's choyce for succesfully extracapsularly treated cataract. It may be inserted also as a primary procedure. This then is the same as the transiridectomy safety clip iris medallion lens of Fig. 13. However, in case of a larger incision the lens of Fig. 13 is preferred. For surgical technique, see Fig. 15.

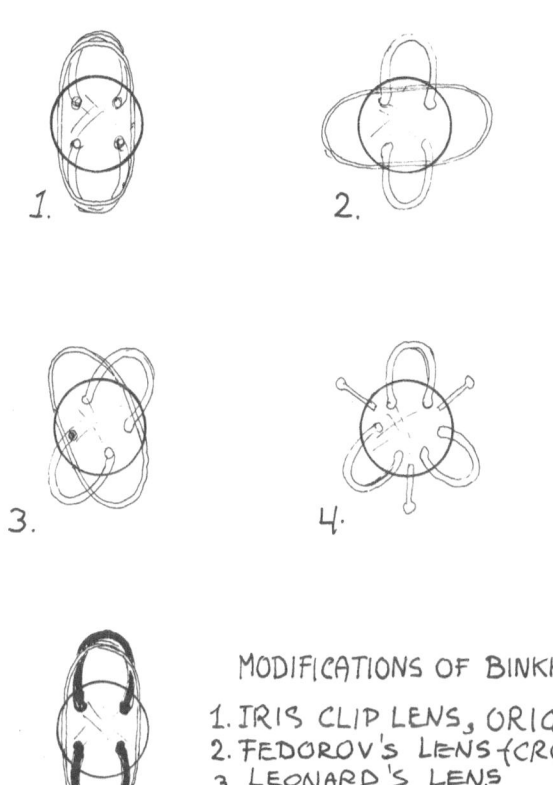

MODIFICATIONS OF BINKHORST's

1. IRIS CLIP LENS, ORIGINAL.
2. FEDOROV's LENS (CROSSED)
3. LEONARD'S LENS
4. FEDOROV'S "SPUTNIK" LENS
5. BINKHORST'S BLACK POS-
   TERIOR LOOP LENS.

Fig. 11

Fig. 15.

Fig. 15 is the 'iris medallion lens' sutured to the iris. This lens has been used in several hundred cases over a period of 6 years. An iris suture is taking care of lens fixation. The mode of action of this suture is not to suture the lens to the iris but only to keep it in contact with the upper iris border. (see Fig. 16A; 16B.)

Fig. 16.

On dilatation the iris medallion lens will move upwards with the pupil border producing a partially phakic and partially aphakic pupil, See: Physiological optics of pseudophakia. (in preparation).

This has little influence on visual acuity. It must be stressed that the position of the suture is critical. If placed too high the lens may ride against the cornea. If placed too low its function to prevent luxation may fail. The surgical technique will be described elsewhere. Note, that the suture is buried under the haptic flange of the lens. The construction of the iris

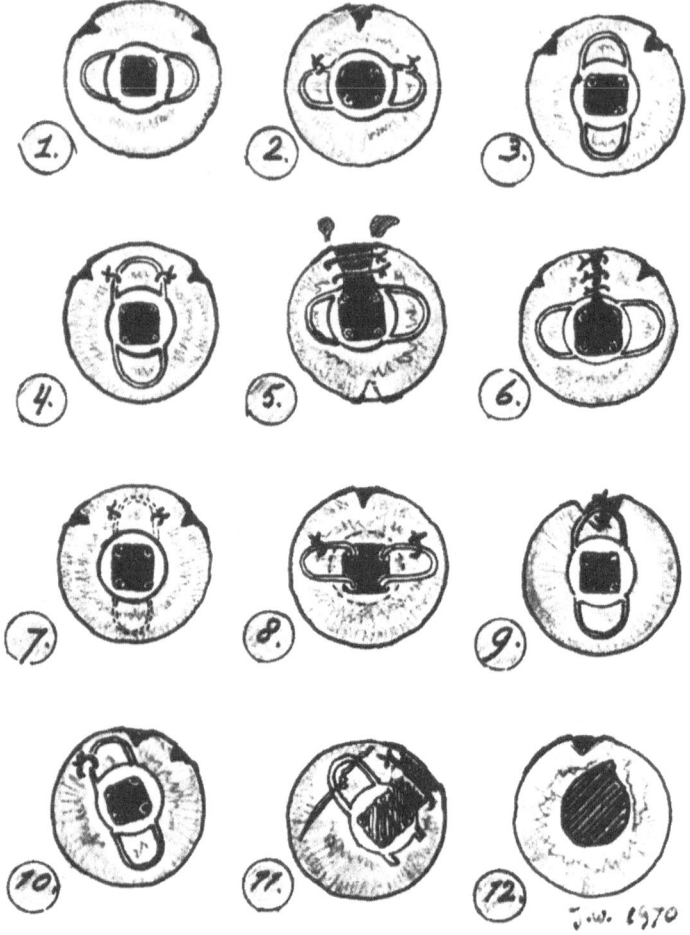

Fig. 12

medallion lens: It has the standard type of optical central portion. An excentric haptic ring has been added. This excentric haptic part has a stabilizing function. Furthermore by this construction the smallest possible horizontal diameter has been obtained, which effectively prevents the 'intermittent corneal touch syndrome' leading to corneal dystrophy. The basic construction of the iris medallion lens has been used in various modifications.

Fig. 17.

As it has been noted that under certain circumstances the perlon iris suture may break mechanically or may become absorbed the suturing technique has been changed. Steel sutures are now used instead of perlon as a transiridectomy fixation method. Fig. 18 is showing one design of lens made for steel fixation. As the steel sutures are too rigid for intraocular knotting a

82

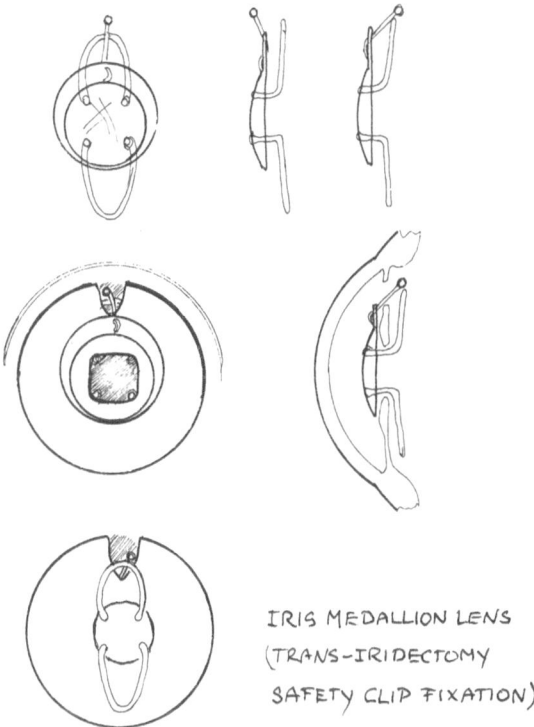

IRIS MEDALLION LENS
(TRANS-IRIDECTOMY
SAFETY CLIP FIXATION)

Fig. 13

different way of suture closure is used. Small slots have been made in the lens through which the steel suture can be bent. The final configuration of this type of iris suture resembles a simple staple.

Great care must be taken here to bend the sutures flat with the lens surface. For details on the surgical technique of stainless steel iris suturing see: Surgical technique of iris medallion lens. Note, that the iris medallion lens in its modification for steel fixation suture is directly derived from the original iris medallion lens. The necessary slots in the lens can be easily cut by the surgeon himself with a pair of fine scissors.

A further modification of the steel fixation suture lens is a lens with two special slots for suture passage which have been oriented outward and in which two more notches have been added in order to bury the free ends of the steel suture under the lens.

In this type of suture fixation the steel suture is kept stretched and no stapling is required.

Fig. 18.

The metal parts of the iris medallion lens are made of titanium or platinum. Platinum is good material for making the transiridectomy clips, as the platinum is highly flexible. The titanium however shows interesting mechanical properties as well. It has a higher resilience and it is harder to bend.

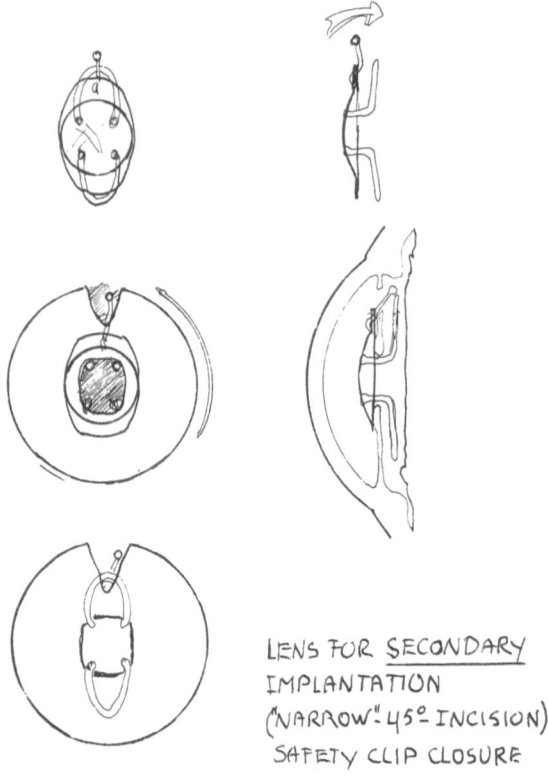

LENS FOR SECONDARY
IMPLANTATION
("NARROW" 45° INCISION)
SAFETY CLIP CLOSURE

Fig. 14

Different types of lenses have been designed by using titanium as the basic material for loops and clips of various types. A typical example is Fig. 19: the iris medallion lens of the 'scarabee' type. This lens has two sharp prongs which are inserted directly through the iris stroma and make contact with the single posterior loop. This lens is only advocated in case of extracapsular lensextraction, in view of the sharpness of the prongs which otherwise may damage the anterior vitreous surface. For consequences of anterior vitreous damage: See: Lensimplantation and macular degeneration. (in preparation).

This lens is shown as an example of trans stromal fixation. It is not recommanded as a routine type of lens.

Fig. 19.

Is showing the same as Fig. 18 with a different application: The insertion of a lens prior to lensextraction. This type of insertion has been succesfully tried but is not recommended as a routine procedure either because corneal contact during lensextraction cannot effectively be prevented in case of a shallow anterior chamber during surgery.

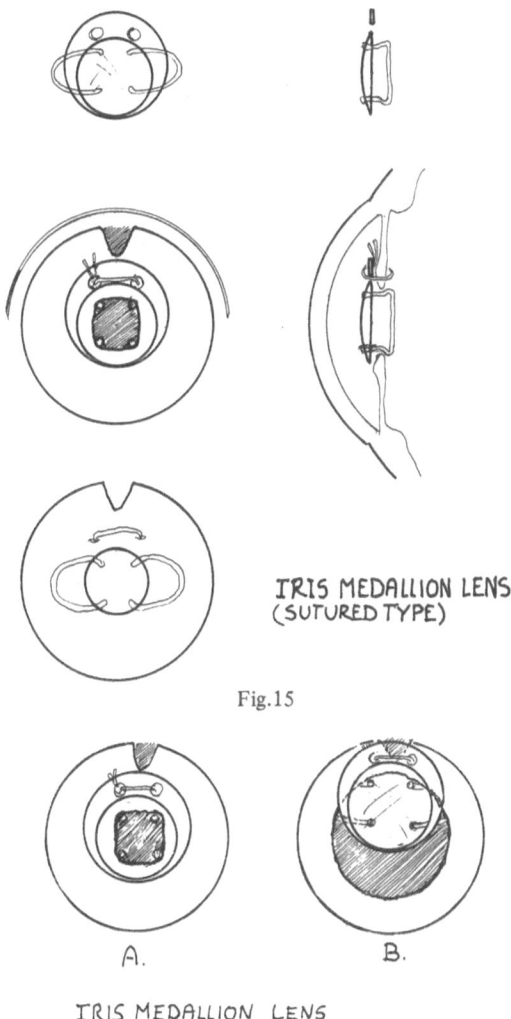

IRIS MEDALLION LENS
(SUTURED TYPE)

Fig.15

A.   B.

IRIS MEDALLION LENS
A.   CONSTRICTED PUPIL
B.   DILATED PUPIL

Fig. 16

Fig. 20.

Shows a prototype of a so-called single posterior loop lens. It has transiridectomy fixation. The single posterior loop is joined to the anterior haptic part in which a hole has been made. Insertion of this lens is extremely simple but the application of the suture may be difficult.

The ring clip fixation is performed with a miniature staple made of platinum. This part of the surgical procedure proved too difficult for general use.

The series of lenses discussed in this paper have been designed to find the

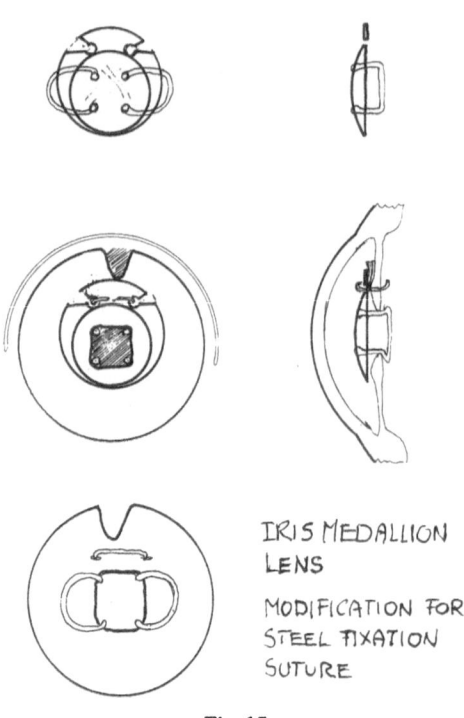

IRIS MEDALLION
LENS

MODIFICATION FOR
STEEL FIXATION
SUTURE

Fig. 17

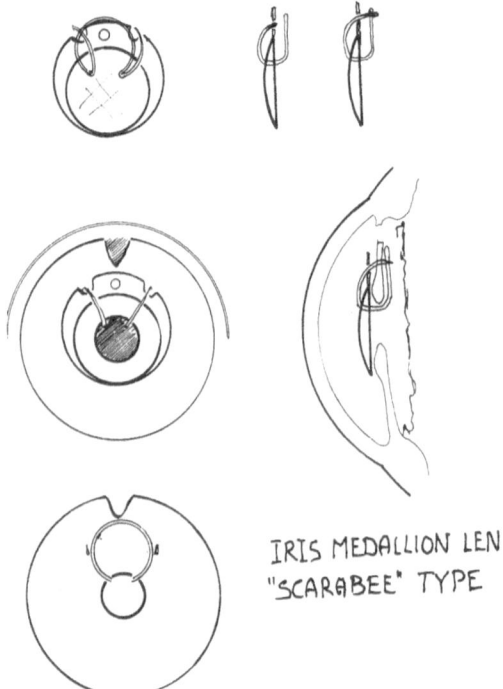

IRIS MEDALLION LEN
"SCARABEE" TYPE

Fig. 18

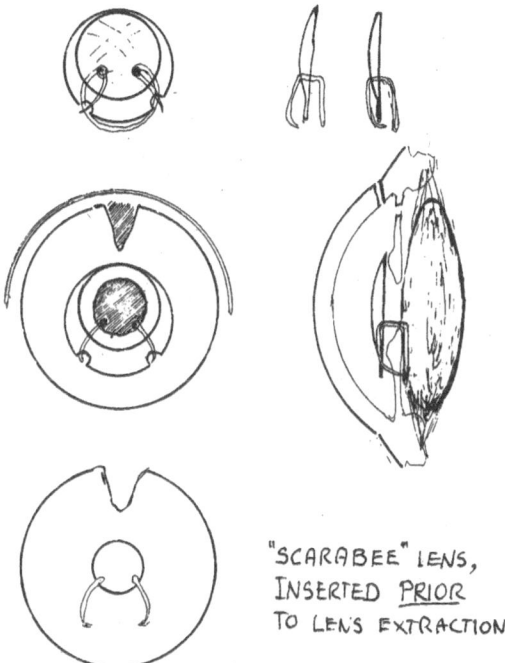

"SCARABEE" LENS,
INSERTED PRIOR
TO LENS EXTRACTION

Fig. 19

mechanically simplest lens which gives the maximum of safety in terms of absence of contact with intraocular structures and 'unluxatability'. It must be stressed that, though all of these lenses have been tried, none of these 'trials' have been of a truly experimental nature. Any of the demonstrated fixation procedures is effective but they greatly differ in their ease of application.

Fig. 21.

A further example of a transiridectomy closure.

This lense has preplaced steel suture fixed to the posterior loop. This suture is passed through the iridectomy and clamped in a notch in the anterior haptic part. Only one case had been performed with this type of suture. In view of the development of easier transiridectomy clip procedures this lens has also be abandoned.

Fig. 22.

It occurred to us that the transiridectomy principle could also be built into the posterior loop. In the case demonstrated the posterior loop has a special hook which by its resilience (titanium) will clip itself around the anterior haptic portion.

This is a technically very succesfull lens but the clip as such is vulnerable and may become distorted in unexperienced hands. This has been a reason to discard this principle.

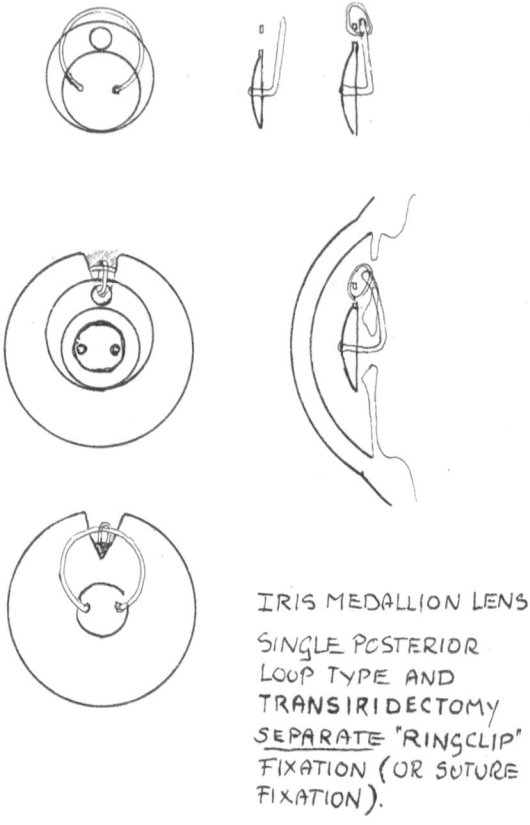

IRIS MEDALLION LENS

SINGLE POSTERIOR
LOOP TYPE AND
TRANSIRIDECTOMY
SEPARATE "RINGCLIP"
FIXATION (OR SUTURE
FIXATION).

Fig. 20

Fig. 23.

Shows the 'scarabee' lens inserted in the posterior chamber. The anterior loops are the only supporting element. These anterior loops perforate the iris stroma and are embedded in two holes in the haptic rim. This fixation is very satisfactory but from the surgical point of view this procedure proved technically exacting, nevertheless it seems that this posterior chamber fixation with this form of trans stromal fixation, in combination with extracapsular surgery may lead to an efficient system of lens fixation.

Fig. 24

Fig. 24 shows a modification of the steel suture transiridectomy closure in which the steel suture is preplaced on the posterior loop. The special notches in the haptic rim B serve for fixation of the steel transiridectomy clip. This type of lens is extremely easy to insert and to fixate.

Unfortunately the manufacturing process of this type of lens seems too difficult to make it possible to manufacture this type of lens serially. The author has attached a special mallcable stainless steel clip himself.

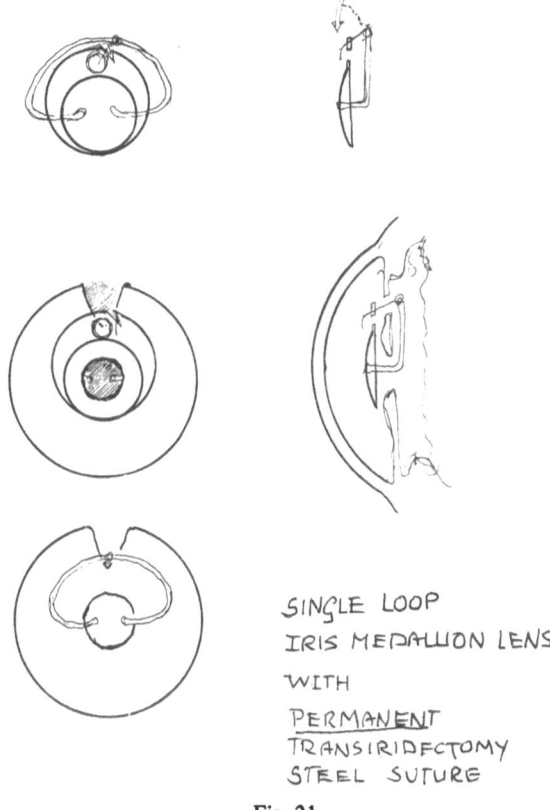

SINGLE LOOP
IRIS MEDALLION LENS
WITH
PERMANENT
TRANSIRIDECTOMY
STEEL SUTURE

Fig. 21

Fig. 25.

In cases of extracapsular extraction a large single posterior loop artificial lens has been used. To improve fixation a transiridectomy stainless steel suture has been attached to the posterior loop in the manner of Fig. 24.

Serial manufacture of this lens is also too difficult and the lens is too vulnerable to mechanical deformation.

In the course of lensdevelopment this lens however has served the useful function of determining the optimal size of a metal posterior loop in terms of mechanical stability.

Fig. 26.

Further studies have been made to determine the optimal type of transiridectomy safety clip closure. Each of the types of closure as illustrated in Fig. 26 were mechanically satisfactory. Only the type of fixation under 1. (the flexible hook) proved surgically acceptable, because sufficient space must remain between the lens and the supporting posterior loop. As the loops shown in 2,3,4 and 5 have some form of mechanical extension to it, there is some chance of damaging the vitreous surface or the posterior

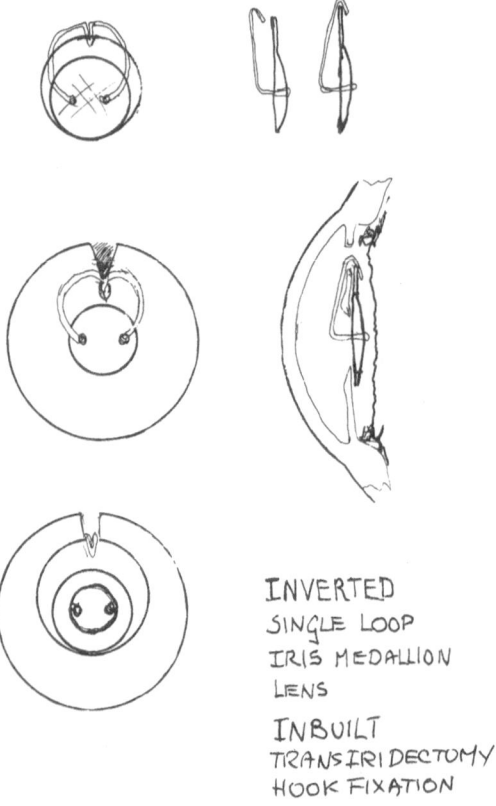

INVERTED
SINGLE LOOP
IRIS MEDALLION
LENS

INBUILT
TRANSIRIDECTOMY
HOOK FIXATION

Fig. 22

pigment layer. Only the lens of fig. 1 has been used extensively. The technique for insertion of this lens is described under: Surgical technique for the single loop safety clip iris medallion lens. It is the author's belief that this lens may replace the author's sutured iris medallion lens, for a number of reasons. *1.* Its insertion is easier than any of the lenses designed. *2.* Transiridectomy clip closure, on condition that the correct technique is used is relatively simple. *3.* The lens is unluxatable on condition that the position and the closure of the transiridectomy clip are applied correctly. *4.* The pupil size of this lens is the smallest of all lenses designed. This results in a reduced photophobia. *5.* This lens can be used in a wide variety conditions, both intra- and extracapsulary.

Fig. 27.

Fig. 27 gives details of the transiridectomy safety clip closure of the single loop iris medallion lens.

Note, that the clip is opened before insertion and should be depressed somewhat to come in contact with the posterior loop. The posterior loop is than lifted over the safety clip loop. The normal resilience of the posterior loop will engage this loop permanently in the transiridectomy hook. The

90

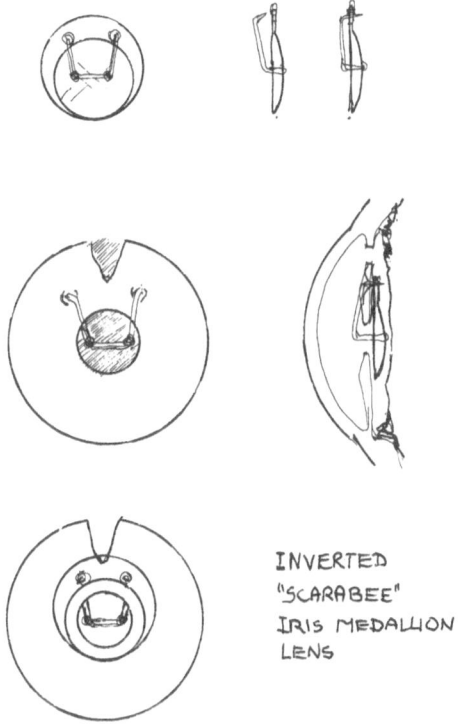

INVERTED
"SCARABEE"
IRIS MEDALLION
LENS

Fig. 23

posterior loop is made of titanium. The transiridectomy safety clip is also made of titanium.

Fig. 28

Some details of the surgical technique of insertion of the lens for secondary implantation: The narrow incision safety clip closure iris medallion lens. After making a 45° temporal incision the lens is placed with its posterior loops behind the iris. In case of an iridectomy being present at 12 o'clock the lens can be rotated intraocularly with the technique as illustrated. When the clip is positioned over the iridectomy internal support with a special spatula and external action with pressure with an iris muscle hook is the least traumatic way to close the safety clip. Rotation of the lens inside th eye is performed with two canula's.

SLOTTED IRIS MEDALLION LENS.

Fig. 29.

By adding one slot to the right perforation of the haptic rim it is possible to insert this iris medallion lens with stainless steel suture fixation. See: Surgical technique of iris medallion lens.

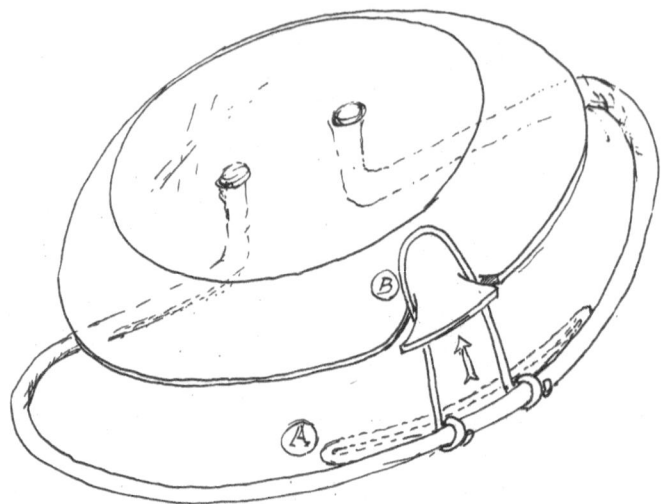

CONSTRUCTION OF
READY-MADE TRANSIRIDECTOMY
CLOSURE
(A): FOLDED
(B): EXTENDED, AND CLIPPED
TO HAPTIC EDGE OF IRIS
MEDALLION LENS.

Fig. 24

Fig. 30.

Surgical details of insertion of a slotted iris medallion lens.

Note, the straight stainless steel suture is already present in the iris.

The slot is in the left hole. Generally a right hole is slotted as this is technically easier for a right handed surgeon.

SUMMARY

Description of a number of artificial lenses and a discussion of their various merits and disadvantages.

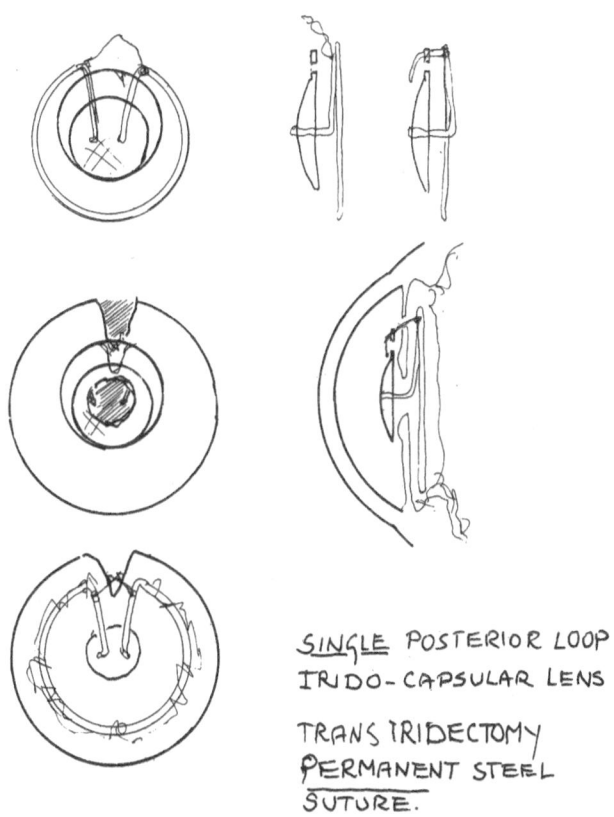

SINGLE POSTERIOR LOOP
IRIDO-CAPSULAR LENS

TRANS IRIDECTOMY
PERMANENT STEEL
SUTURE.

Fig. 25

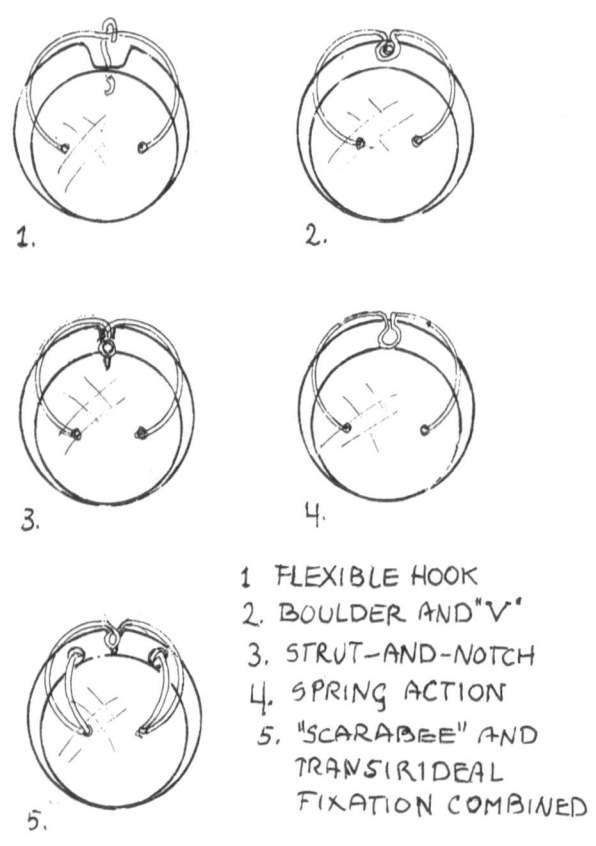

1 FLEXIBLE HOOK
2. BOULDER AND "V"
3. STRUT-AND-NOTCH
4. SPRING ACTION
   5. "SCARABEE" AND
      TRANSIRIDEAL
      FIXATION COMBINED

VARIATIONS FOR TRANSIRIDEAL FIXATION
OF SINGLE LOOP IRIS MEDALLION LENS

Fig. 26

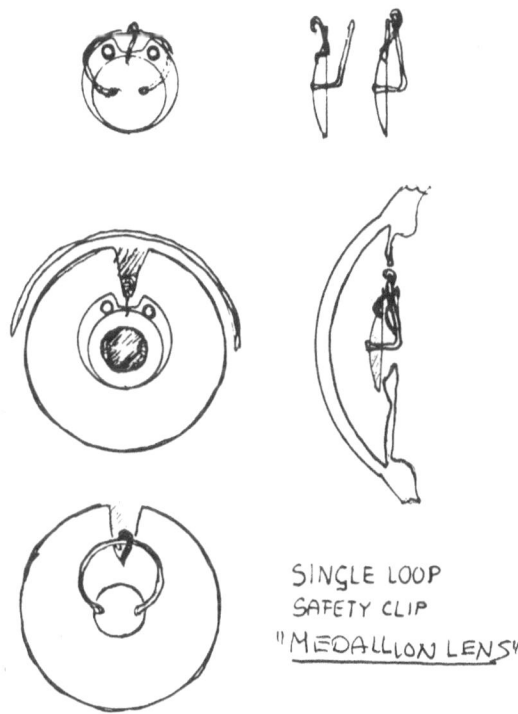

SINGLE LOOP
SAFETY CLIP
"MEDALLION LENS"

Fig. 27

95

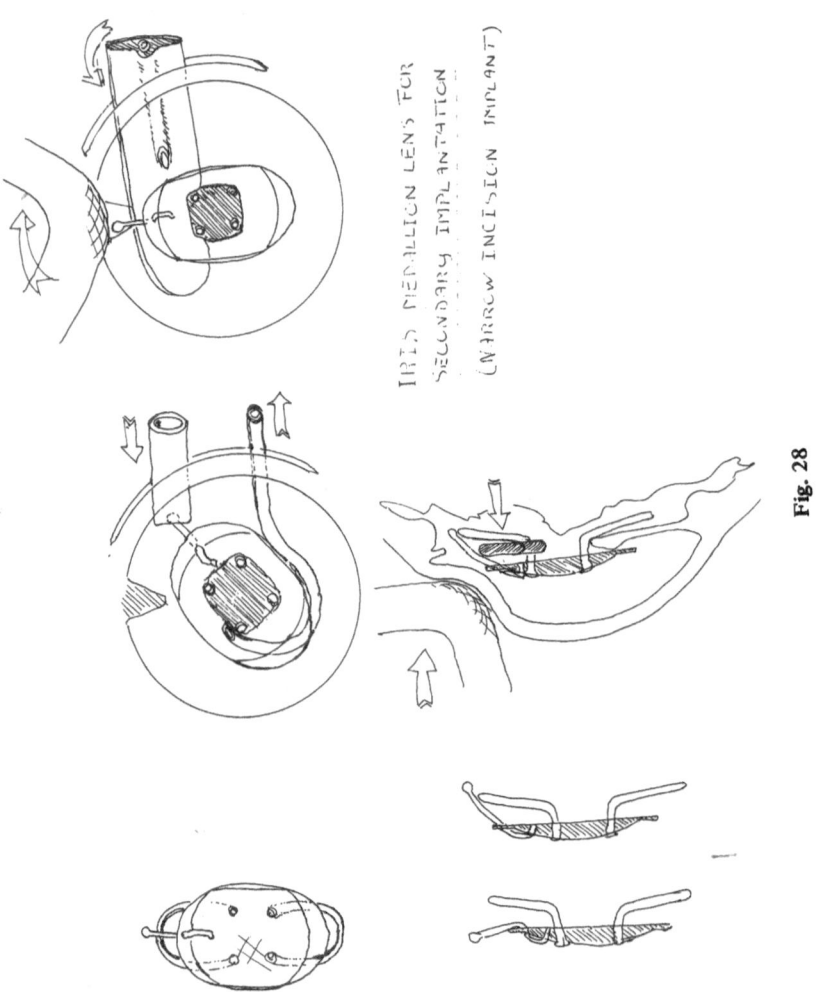

IRIS MEDALLION LENS FOR
SECONDARY IMPLANTATION
(NARROW INCISION IMPLANT)

Fig. 28

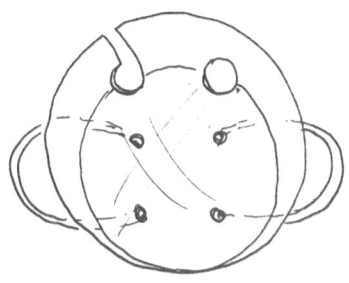

IRIS MEDALLION LENS
SLOTTED TYPE, FOR
STAINLESS STEEL
SUTURE FIXATION.

Fig. 29

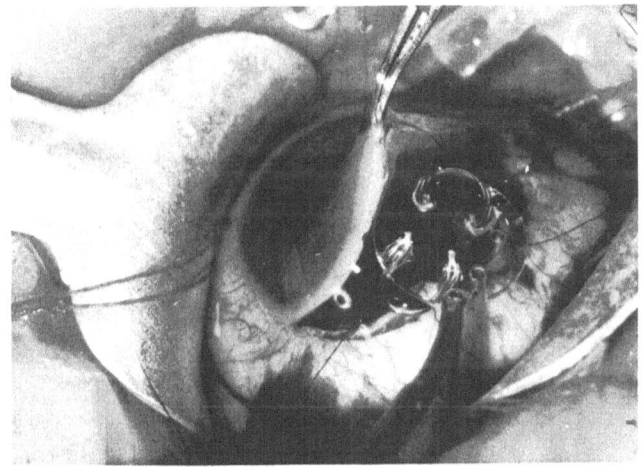

Fig. 30

REFERENCE

BINKHORST C.D. Transactions American Academy of Ophthalmology and Otolaryngology (September-October 1973) The iridocapsular (two-loop)lens and the iris-clip (four-loop) lens in pseudophakia.

Author's address:
J.G.F. Worst
Dept. of Ophthalmology
Refaja Hospital
Stadskanaal
The Netherlands

97

SOME THOUGHTS ON THE FIXATION
OF INTRAOCULAR LENSES

C.D. BINKHORST

(Terneuzen)

INTRODUCTION

It can readily be understood that a personal experience of lens implant surgery of nearly twenty years has put one to thinking on several aspects of this fascinating and promising kind of surgery. Apart from its surgical approach, the fixation of the intraocular lens, -and with that its design-, has turned out to be of the utmost importance for the result and especially for the long-term fate of the eye. Whereas surgery can not really be learned from a script, the many aspects of fixation lend itself to description much better (BINKHORST, 1973).

Lens implants in the eye are in a much more favourable position compared with many types of implants elsewhere in the body. The latter having mostly extensive contact with surrounding tissues, lens implants can be placed in a completely or nearly completely humoral environment. This may well be the secret of the good tolerance of the eye for intraocular lens implants and of the durability of the material. A humoral environment helps to protect the tissues of the eye from being damaged by the implant and protects the implant from being desintegrated by the same tissues. From the foregoing it will be clear that if there has to be any contact between lens implant and eye, this contact should be limited to the utmost. For fixation purposes the apparent choice is between the epithelium – and endothelium – lined iris membrane without perforating it, and the avascular and acellular capsular membrane. Thus the basic surgical technique may be the intracapsular as well as the extracapsular technique of cataract extraction and the present principle of fixation of an intraocular lens is membrane fixation.

The possibility of dislocation of an intraocular lens was and is looked upon as one of the shortcomings of lens implant treatment. The rather common practice however to remove the implant from the eye, once it had been dislocated, was not at all justified. Repositioning of the lens as has been described elsewhere, nearly always would have been an easy procedure and very rarely would have turned out to be impossible.

It has been said that the efficiency of the fixation of an artificial lens is inferior to the fixation of the crystalline lens as far as injuries are concerned. In my experience this has not been proven to be correct. Adequate fixation of an intraocular lens can stand as much trauma as the zonular fixation of the crystalline, though both of them may give way (Fig. 1). As to 'spontaneous' dislocation, these have been overcome nearly completely to-day.

99

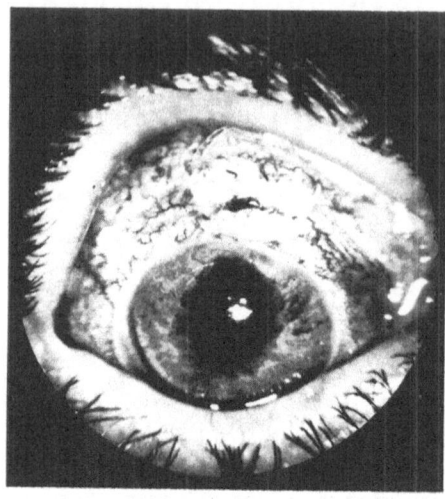

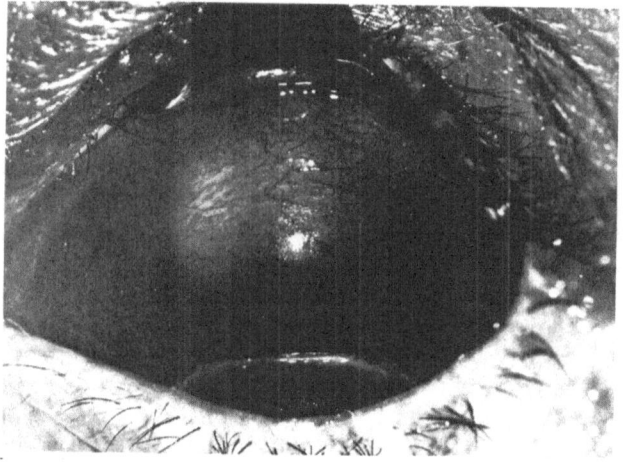

Fig. 1 a. Intercalar rupture of the sclera with subconjunctival dislocation of an artificial lens. (Courtesy H. HIRSCHMAN, M.D.).
b. Idem with subconjunctival dislocation of the crystalline lens.

Reviewing past experiences, as well personal and from others, it can be said that anterior dislocations were much more dangerous than posterior dislocations, especially when not noticed early (figs. 2,3). As to the first the corneal endothelium would suffer. As to the latter it seems that posterior dislocation of an artificial lens even into the vitreous has less consequences for the eye. It has been said that somewhere in the world, there is a patient who does very well with two artificial lenses, one in the proper place and one in the vitreous.

HISTORY

On the 29th November 1949 the first intraocular lens has been inserted by Harold Ridley (Ridley, 1951). He seemed convinced that 'the proper place

100

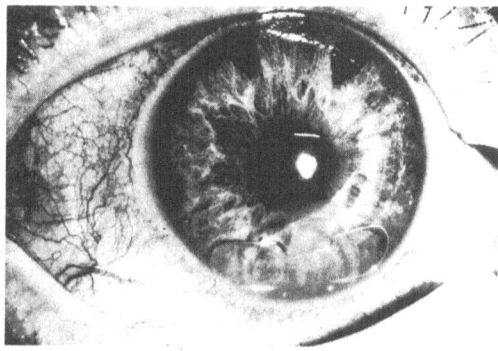

Fig. 2. Anterior dislocation of an artificial lens, diagnosed only six weeks after its onset. Corneal oedema not subsiding after repositioning of the lens.

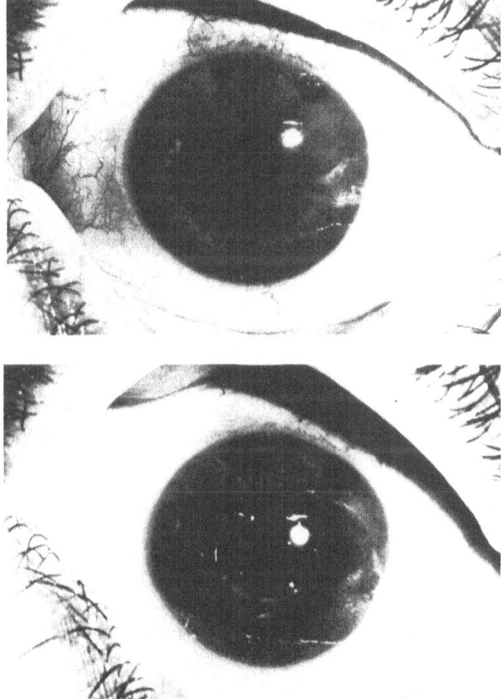

Fig. 3 a. Posterior dislocation of an artificial lens.
b. Same eye with dilated pupil. The body of the lens turns out to be well-centered. The dislocation never raised any problem.

for an artificial lenticulus must surely be where Nature intended the crystalline to be', viz. in the posterior chamber. Though in several cases he relied on the vitreous face for support without success, inserting his lens after intracapsular extraction, the majority of lenses were inserted after extracapsular extraction. His method of fixation uses both the iris and the posterior capsule of the crystalline, — strenghtened as it would be later with the formation of a capsular membrane —, as its support and is irido-capsular fixation. Very often it must have remained obscure what happened with the posterior capsula and its zonular fibers during insertion of the bulky Ridley lens and in many eyes potential dislocation into the vitreous must have been inserted with the lens itself. However, according to my own experience, with the posterior capsula and the zonular fibers undamaged, even the heavy Ridley lens would stay in place, finally sticking to the capsular membrane

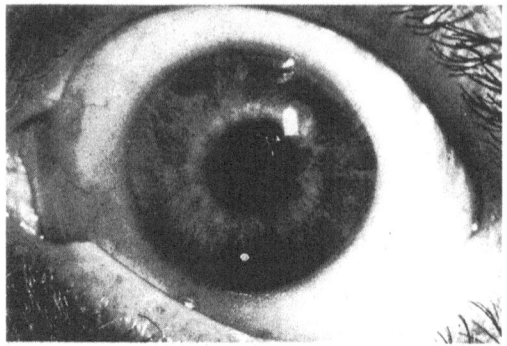

Fig. 4. Original Ridley-lens, some 20 years after implantation.

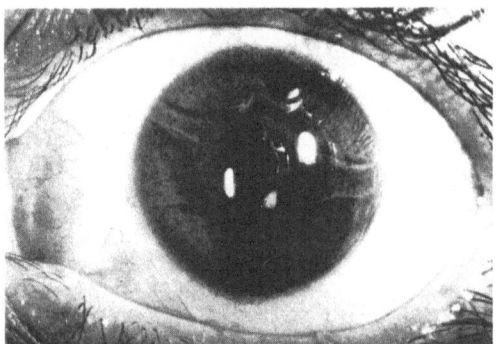

Fig. 5. Schreck's chamber angle supported lens, one of the few eyes that did not develop corneal dystrophy.

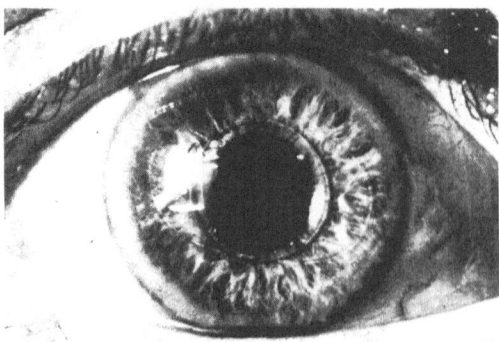

Fig. 6. One of the first eyes with four-loop iris clip lens. Note the original horizontal position of the lens.

(Fig. 4). Though EPSTEIN (1959) improved the Ridley lens with several modifications this type of membrane or irido-capsular fixation soon was abandoned and only regained interest some ten years later, though with different lens designs.

Subsequently the anterior chamber has been selected as a place for the lens. BARON (1953) speculated about a lens floating in the anterior chamber without any touch at all, – 'l'ideal serait d'avoir des lentilles flottantes dans l'humeur aqueuse' –. Recognizing that this was utopia he himself and many others promptly chose the delicate angle area with the adjacent corneal endothelium for support, with rigid or with elastic support, without or with transscleral anchoring of the lens. Angle-supported lenses generally became known as the Strampelli-type of lens (STRAMPELLI, 1954). It seems unbelievable to-day that the inventors of angle-supported lenses and those who followed them, including myself, have been so little endothelial-minded as to believe that the immediate good results would last a life-time. This holds especially true for those lenses with badly shaped and badly polished supports (Fig. 5). It is Choyce's merit (CHOICE, 1970) to have proven that with really sophisticated supports the corneal endothelium could be avoided to the ut-most and consequently the incidence of endothelial and corneal breakdown could be lowered in a significant way.

In the meanwhile and independently EPSTEIN (1959) and the author (BINKHORST, 1959) started to pioneer on the iris diaphragm as a support for the lens. SCHILLINGER (1958) and co-workers did experiments on animals. EPSTEIN inserted the first iris-fixated lens, the so-called collar stud lens after intracapsular extraction, as far back as 1953 and only reported about it in 1959.

The author developped his so-called iris clip lens in 1957 and has been using it in the human eye since august 1958 (Fig. 6). To-day the iris clip lens is still principally the same lens. Only minor changes on the shape and the length of the loops and on the loop insertions were carried out in the course of years (BINKHORST, 1973). EPSTEIN (1959), after he had abandonned the collar stud principle, developped the so called Maltese cross lens, a pupillary plane lens, at first with solid and later with fenestrated supports. A modification of this lens was adopted on a larger scale in the U.S. first by GALIN and later by JAFFE and the Miami Group under the name Copeland lens or iris plane lens. The iris clip lens and its modifications being prepupillary lenses and the Maltese cross lens and its derivations being pupillary or iris plane lenses. The extreme importance of this difference should be pointed out, this importance hiding in the extent of tissue contact and in the possibility of communication between the anterior and the posterior chamber of the eye (Fig. 7).

The iris clip lens and its modification the capsular lens are lenses with four respectively two loops, the lens body and the posterior loops being on a different level. The lensbody is in a prepupillary position and free from the pupil. The iris clip lens became widely used, not only in the Netherlands but also in several other countries all over the world. FEDOROV used the iris clip lens for the first time in 1963 in the S.U., but in 1964 started to use a modification of iris clip lens with the anterior and posterior loops at right angles. Since 1968 he is using another modification of iris clip lens with

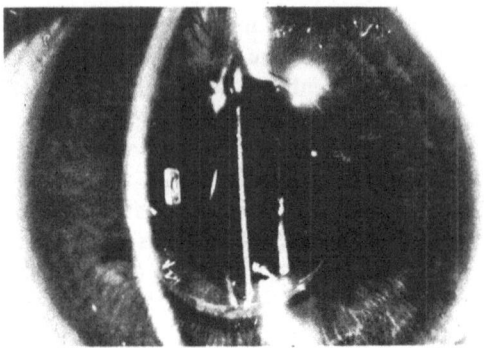

Fig. 7. Two-loop irido-capsular lens. Note the clearance between posterior capsula, iris surface and lens body.

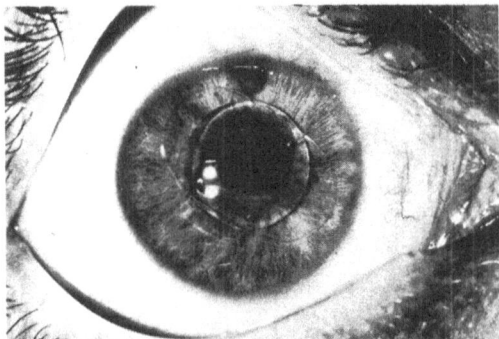

Fig. 8. First four-loop iris clip lens inserted after extracapsular cataract extraction (december 1963).

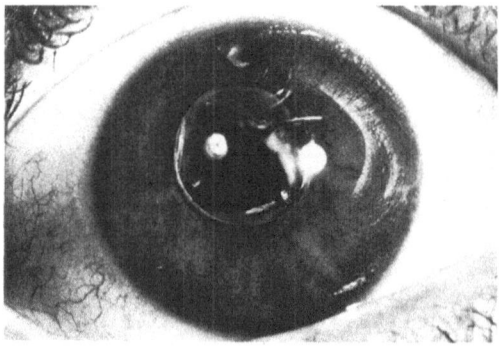

Fig. 9. First two-loop (irido-) capsular lens inserted after extracapsular cataract extraction (september 1965).

three posterior loops and three antenne-like extensions in front of the iris. This lens in our country got the name Spoetnik lens. In order to better distinguish the anterior and posterior loops LEONARD suggested to mount them with a small angle, and LURIE advised the use of black posterior loops. Other iris supported lenses were developped by WORST (1971,) and used on a large scale.

The possibility of capsular support had been forgotten until in December

104

1963 the author inserted an iris clip lens after extracapsular extraction of a traumatic cataract, followed by several others (Fig. 8). The posterior loops got embedded in adhesions between iris and capsular membrane. Lenses thus supported could not move around inside the eye. The anterior loops lost their function under these circumstances. On the 16th September 1965 the first lens with only posterior loops was inserted into a traumatic aphakic eye with a capsular membrane (Fig. 9). The posterior loops were inserted between iris and capsular membrane after posterior synechiae had been loosened. Afterwards the loops were firmly embedded in irido-capsular adhesions. This was the origin of the two-loop (irido-) capsular lens (BINK-HORST et al, 1972). FEDOROV during his visit to Terneuzen in 1966, also seemed to have thought about capsular fixation. He stressed the point that the capsular membrane was extremely suitable for fixation as it was an avascular membrane.

THE FURTHER DEVELOPMENT OF IMPLANT SURGERY IN THE NETHERLANDS. PRESENT ROUTINE TECHNIQUES OF THE AUTHOR.

Iris supported lenses.

The normal iris membrane is strong enough to hold a light device such as the iris clip lens and the sphincter muscle is able to keep it centered. The iris membrane and its pupillary opening however represent no stable support, and this for two reasons. a. its changing pupil width. b. its changing position between vitreous body and aqueous humour. Under certain conditions this could give rise to dislocation, to endothelial contact, possibly to 'spontaneous' haemorrhages and likely also to changes of the hydrodynamics in the chambers of the eye.

a, Changing pupil width.

The constricted pupil will keep the lens well-centered, whereas in a dilated pupil the lens can ride in any direction depending on the position of the eye. Riding in the direction of its axis can even lead to anterior or posterior dislocation (Fig. 10). The majority of cases develop iris adhesions, especially of the pupillary margin, with the loop insertions or with the vitreous face and thus dislocation is prevented. We got the impression that this was especially the case after cryo extraction of the cataract and less after forceps extraction (Fig. 11). Worthwhile mentioning in this respect is the verdict of LEONARD that 'the best guarantee against dislocation is a traumatic surgical technique'. In a sense we followed this advice in a few cases and tried to promote iris synechiae by sqeezing the iris with teethed forceps and also by touching it with the cryo-probe. Further light coagulation was through of as possible means to improve fixation.

Yet we had a 15 to 20 percent dislocations in the earlier years and therefore started the prescription of miotics to every patient. With it the incidence of dislocations fell down to almost zero. This however was still not considered the ideal solution as not every patient was using his drops

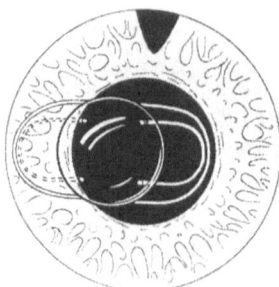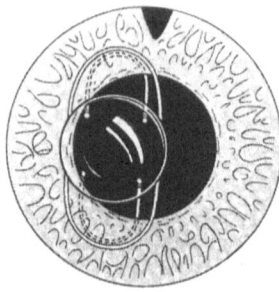

Fig. 10 a. A horizontally placed lens can dislocate when the eye turns sidewards.
b. A vertically placed lens in the same circumstances, can not dislocate.

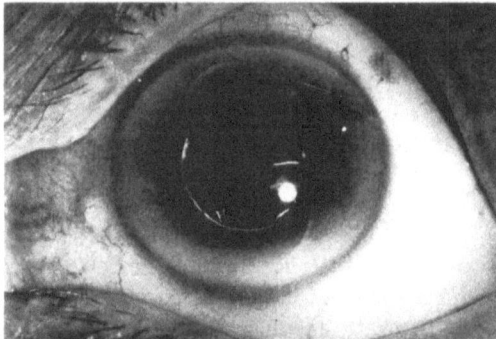

Fig. 11. Synechiae of the upper iris segment after cryo-extraction of the cataract.

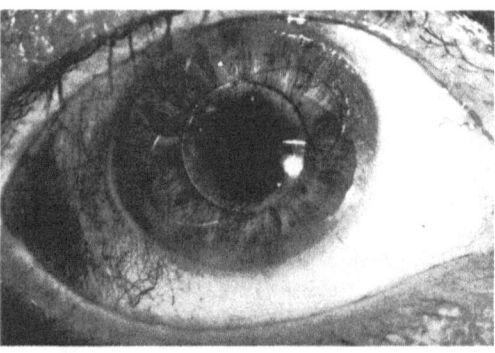

Fig. 12. So-called 'worn-out' pupil after prolonged use of miotics. Local atrophy of the sphincter muscle at the posterior loop insertions.

regularly and as not every pupil reacted correctly. Also the pupillary border was suffering from indentations and atrophy caused by the posterior loop insertions (Fig. 12). Histological studies by MANSCHOT showed amongst other minor pathology of the pupillary border a definite sphincter muscle atrophy in nearly every case (Fig. 13).

It was clear that a reliable method was needed with which we could abandon the regular use of miotics and which would permit full pupil dilatation without fear for dislocation, if nesessary. WORST (1971,) in February

106

Fig. 13. Nearly complete sphincter muscle atrophy after prolonged use of miotics
(courtesy W. MANSCHOT, M.D.).

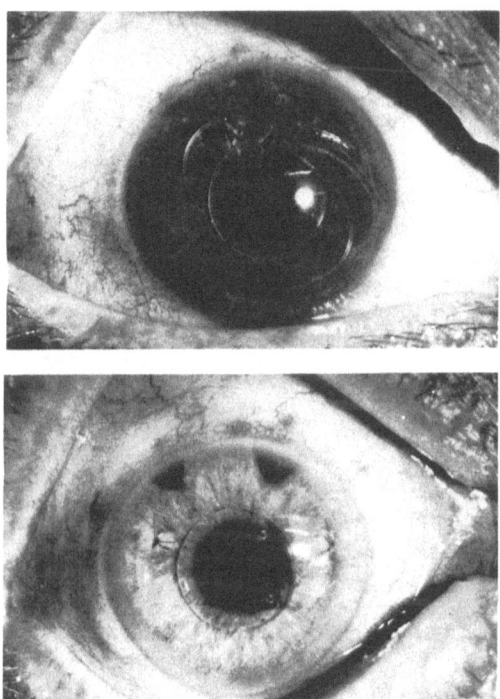

Fig. 14 a. Four-loop iris clip lens. The upper anterior loop is stitched to the iris.
b. Idem. Both anterior loops are stitched to the iris.c

1969 advised to suture the lens on the iris, at first one loop, later the
equatorial zone of the lens body (Fig. 14). This led him to the development
of an enlarged lens body with two holes in the upper segment to pass a
monofilament perlon suture (medallion lens). As of no practical value any
more he suppressed the anterior loops. The author (BINKHORST, 1973) in
March 1970 changed his surgical technique slightly whilst inserting the iris
clip lens in vertical position, and thus being able to connect both upper
loops in a peripheral iris coloboma in the 12 o'clock position with a monofilament perlon suture. If loosely tied the loop suture permits the lens to
remain in the center during pupil dilatation, at least in the upright position,
whereas lenses with iris suture ride high during pupil dilatation (Fig. 15). A
suggestion of using a peripheral coloboma for further fixation of the lens

107

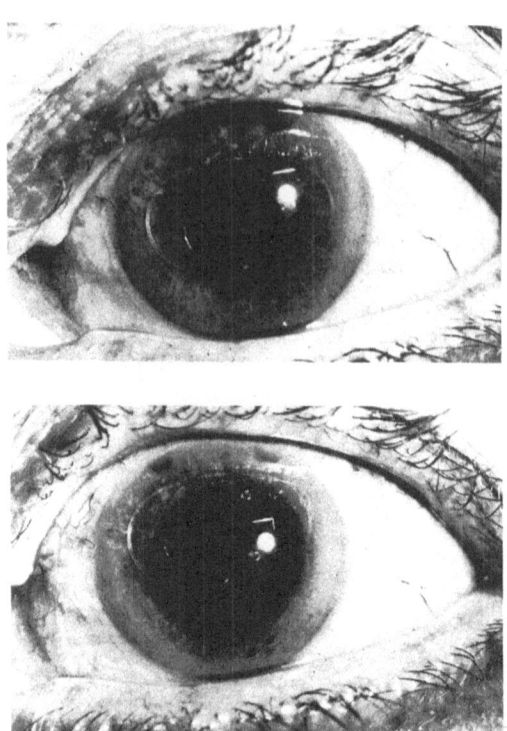

Fig. 14c. Four-loop iris clip lens. The lensbody is stitched to the iris. d. Same eye as Fig. 14c. When the pupil dilates, the lens rides high and may contact the corneal endothelium.

had already been made by RIDLEY in 1956' ... to prevent a lens from slipping downward over the face of the vitreous, e.g. suspension of the lens by a projection hooked into the peripheral iridectomy ...'.

It was however never realized. LEONARD in 1968 realized a modification of one of the anterior loops that would make transiridectomy loop connection possible. It was however never used. In December 1973 WORST announced that he had partially abandonned the iris stitch technique because of unreliability of the perlon. He is developing now a transiridectomy hooking technique with a finger-like extension mounted at the edge of the lens body (safety pin principle).

b. Changing position of the iris between vitreous body and aqueous humour.

Also in another respect the iris membrane in an aphakic eye is an unstable membrane, being subject to fore and aft movements and to tilting movements, dependant on the position of the eye and on its movements (iridodonesis). Also for this reason iris supported lenses are subject to displacement within the eye (pseudophakodonesis). In cases where is only little clearance between lens and corneal endotheliun in the normal position, the lens can touch the endothelium in other positions of the eye and during eye movements, such as during work, whilst reading, and during the night.

108

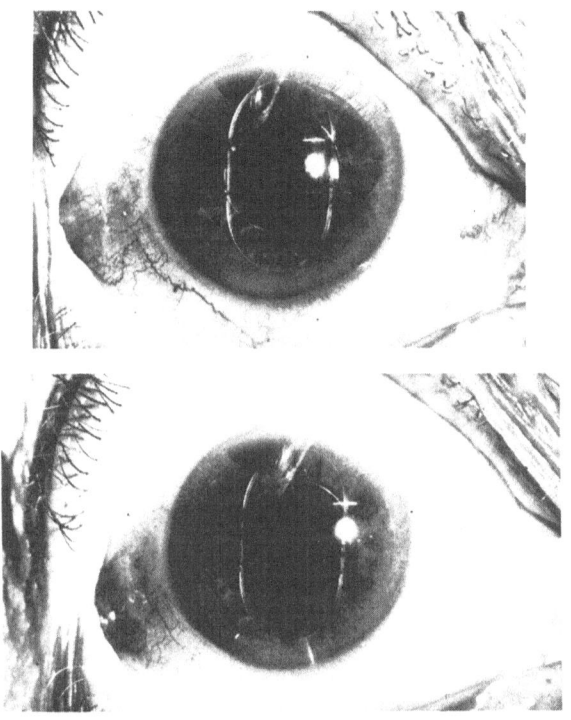

Fig. 15 a. Four-loop iris clip lens. The upper loops are connected with a monofilament perlon suture through the peripheral iris coloboma.
b. Same eye as Fig. 15a. The lens stays centered when the pupil dilates.

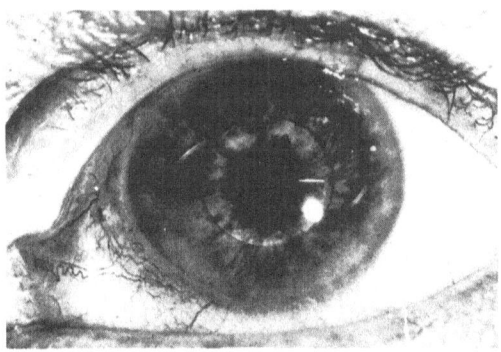

Fig. 16. Four-loop iris clip lens in horizontal position after intracapsular cataract extraction. Contact dystrophy of the cornea at 9 o'clock caused by excessive tilting movements of the lens (pseudophakodonesis).

Gravity and centrifugal forces exert their influence on the lens. Though mostly only after many years, corneal dystrophy can develop by the mechanism of periodical endothelial contact. Whereas in a follow-up study in 1966-1967 we could state a zero percentage of corneal dystrophies after primary implantation in senile cataract, we had to announce a three percent of contact dystrophies in 1972 (BINKHORST, 1973; BINKHORST & LEO-

109

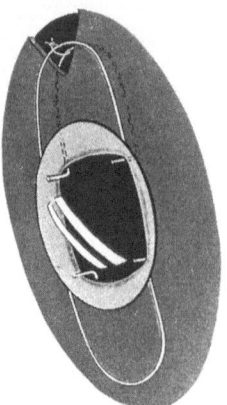

Fig. 17. Transiridectomy loop suture, loosely tied with the lens in vertical position.

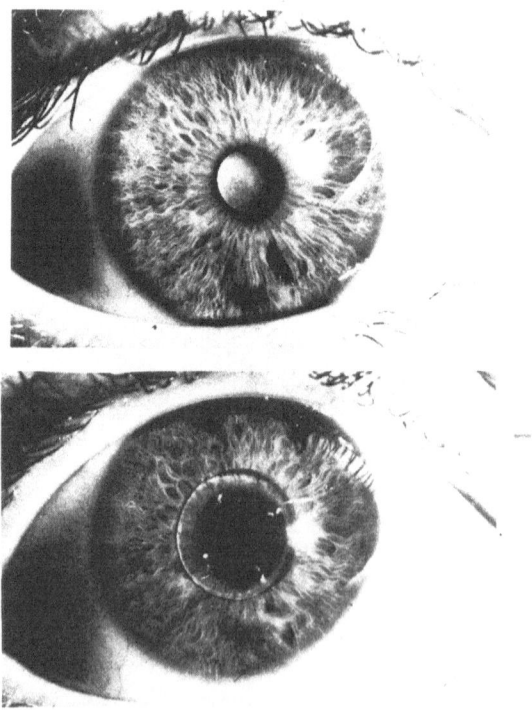

Fig. 18 a. Perforating injury and cataract.
b. Same eye after extracapsular cataract extraction and implantation of a two-loop (irido-) capsular lens.

NARD, 1967). The analysis showed us that in these cases mostly flat anterior loops has been used with an overall length of 9 to 9,5 mm, and that in relatively small and shallow anterior chambers. All lenses showed excessive tilting movements being placed with their axis horizontally (pseudophakodonesis) (Fig. 16). After we had observed displacement of the lens in different positions of the eye, NORDLOHNE (this volume pp. 15-22) could even measure it. Our present technique of iris clip lens implantation after intracapsular cataract extraction successfully aims at the prevention of contact dystrophy, the prevention of dislocation of the lens and at the possibility of a full dilatation of the pupil for fundoscopy without fear of dislocation.

Essential points of this technique are:
1. exact specification of length and curvature of both the anterior and posterior loops.
2. insertion of the lens with its axis vertical
3. additional fixation of the lens with the aid of a transiridectomy loop suture, that should loosely be tied (Fig. 17). In the beginning the application of the loop suture seemed difficult, but with some experience and with the help of a specially designed 12mm long, slightly curved and completely blunt 'needle' threaded with monofilament perlon, it can be done in an easy and atraumatic way. The anterior loop is grasped with a fine forceps whereafter the posterior loop presents itself in the coloboma. The suture is tied over a fine repositor.

In this way both anterior loops are at a comfortable distance from the corneal endothelium, hardly make any tilting movements and it is impossible for the lens to dislocate even when the pupil is dilated to its maximal width.

Capsular supported lenses

Capsular fixation is real immobilization. The lens has a fixed position inside the eye and is not dependent on pupil motility nor is subject to forces of gravity and centrifugation. The weight of the lens is less critical, which allows inert metal loops instead of supramid loops. The contact of the lens with the eye's inner structures is determined. The endothelial clearance remains unchanged. Measurements carried out by NORDLOHNE (this volume pp. 15-22) confirmed this. Moreover the capsular membrane guarantees complete equilibrium inside the eye in the same way as does the crystalline. Later needling in the center of the membrane if necessary does not change this situation basically.

Since 1965 the two-loop (irido) capsular lens gained popularity (BINK-HORST, 1973). It was first used by the author in small eyes (traumatic cataract in children, congenital cataract and some senile cataracts) and later in every type of eye with nearly every type of cataract, either in a one-stage operation or in a two-stage operation (Figs. 18,19,20). Extracapsular cataract extraction with immediate insertion of a two-loop lens is the routine treatment of senile cataract in our Group to-day, the intra-capsular extraction

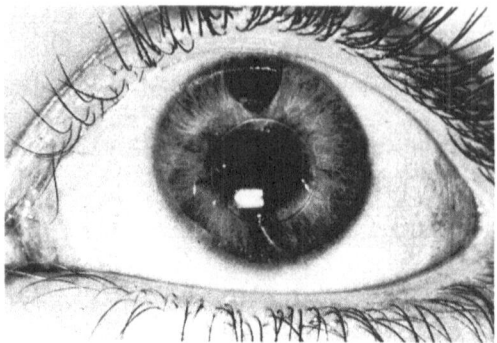

Fig. 19. Unilateral pseudophakia in a five year old boy with bilateral zonular cataracts. Two-loop (irido-) capsular lens.

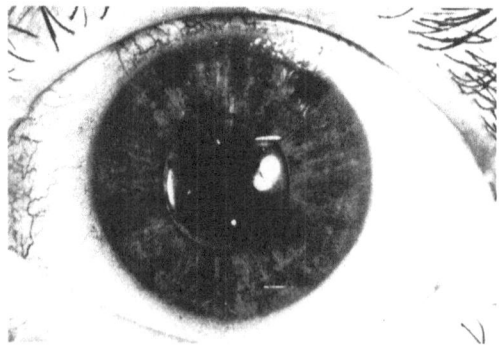

Fig. 20. Pseudophakia after senile cataract. Two-loop (irido-) capsular lens.

with insertion of a four-loop lens being performed on special indications only.

In earlier years miotics were prescribed for several weeks and thus the lens loops became embedded in adhesions between iris and capsular membrane, sometimes to the extent of pupillary seclusion. Most frequent were adhesions of the pupillary border to the capsular membrane or to the loop insertions, rare are flat adhesions to the capsular membrane embedding the posterior loops. In the latter case shrinking processes in the membrane have lead to irregularities of the iris surface, to slight decentration of the lens, to showing of the metal loops through the iris and in a rare case to the formation of iris cysts. Our attitude towards iris involvement however changed in the course of years, which implies now a minimal use of miotics, even of mydriatics. Predominant or even more capsular fixation has taken the place of irido-capsular fixation. The aim is good viz. capsular fixation of the lens with the possibility of as full pupil dilatation as possible. Pupil dilatation is clearly improving with improved postsurgical technique. The ideal dilatation pattern is the wide and round pupil (Fig. 21).

Combatting iris adhesions asks for careful and individual pupil constriction and dilatation policy, which has to be elucidated further.

After removal of as large a piece of anterior capsula as possible with Grieshaber teethed capsular forceps the contents of the capsular bag are

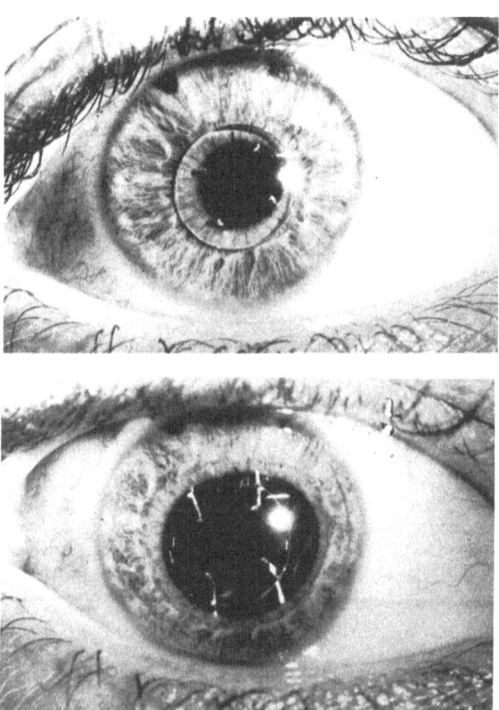

Fig. 21 a. Two-loop (irido-) capsular lens after senile cataract.
b. Same eye with dilated pupil. There is firm capsular fixation of the lens, but no involvement of the iris.

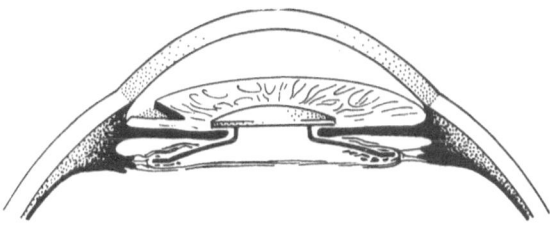

Fig. 22. Two-loop (irido-)capsular lens after extracapsular lens removal. The loops meet cortex remnants at the lens equator. Note the physiological depth of the posterior chamber.

either aspirated and rinsed or expressed and rinsed. The lens loops are supposed to meet some cortical material left at the equatorial zone which later forms a ring-like reinforcement of the posterior capsule that firmly holds the lens loops, whereas the center of the capsula should be as clear as possible (Fig. 22). The relative difficulty of cleaning the upper segment of the capsular bag is solved with the aid of a specially curved irrigation canula (BINKHORST, 1973). During rinsing of the capsular bag one should not too much insist on cleaning the equatorial zone, which anyhow seems to be more or less impossible, even with the new suction and irrigation methods. The patient leaves the operation theatre with 0,25 percent eserine ointment and during the first 72 hours 2 percent pilocarpine eye drops are instilled three times daily. In this way the lens is immobilized and given the opportunity to adhere to the capsular bag. Thereafter miotics are discontinued and the behaviour of the lens studied with the slit-lamp. The already adhering lens remains central if the pupil dilates, otherwise it will ride down. In the first case the pupil is intensively and periodically dilated

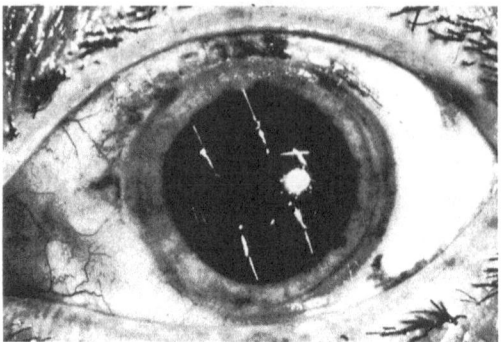

Fig. 23. Two-loop capsular lens on the fourth postoperative day. Pupil dilatation shows the lens adhering in the capsular bag without iris involvement.

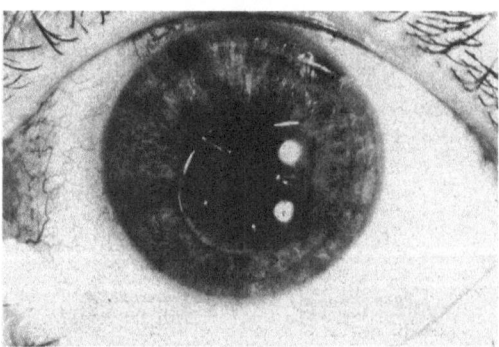

Fig. 24. Two-loop capsular lens on the fourth postoperative day. The lens rides down when the pupil dilates. Miotics have to be continued for another week and the examination repeated.

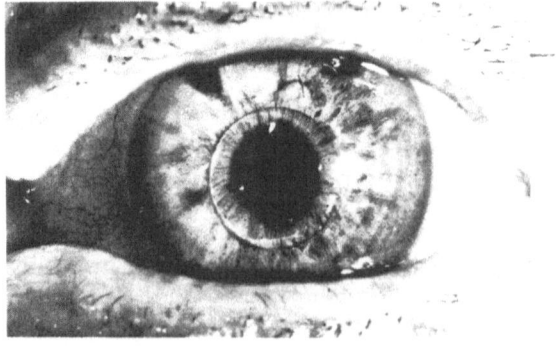

Fig. 25. Two-loop capsular lens without capsular adhesions. The upper loop is stitched to the iris (Binkhorst-Mc Cannell technique).

114

in order to loosen and to prevent iris adhesions (Fig. 23) and in the latter case miotics are instilled for another week and than the procedure is repeated(Fig. 24). Postoperative treatment is a gambling game with capsular fixation and prevention of iris adhesions to win.

In the presence of capsular adhesions iris involvement is of no value for the actual fixation. In a few cases however the lens does not stick to the capsular membrane, but is kept in place by sphincter muscle or by mere iris adhesions. These cases could be responsible for the few exceptions in NORD-LOHNE's series (this volume pp. 15-22) showing different anterior chamber depth in different positions. In rare cases neither capsular nor iris adhesions form. In this respect cataracts with more or less liquefied cortex are suspect (milky cataract). If this is anticipated therefore, a four loop lens secured with a transiridectomy loop suture, should be used according to the intracapsular technique. If the lack of adhesions has not been anticipated, the two-loop lens can be kept in place with miotics or one of its loops can be fixed to the iris with a monofilament perlon suture (Fig. 25).

The technique is as follows (BINKHORST-MC CANNELL): A small corneal incision is made over the underlying loop. The incision should be just wide enough to let pass a fine blunt iris hook. The anterior chamber is evacuated. With an atraumatic needle threaded with perlon the iris and the underlying loop are picked up through the incision (Fig. 26). Then the needle is passed through the cornea in the neighbourhood of the incision and subsequently its perlon is fetched back through the incision with a small blunt iris hook. The suture is loosely tied and cut. Iris and suture are removed from the incision by pushing the lens loop backwards and the incision closed with one perlon stitch. Deepening of the anterior chamber with Ringer solution.

THE PATHOLOGICAL ANTERIOR SEGMENT

Thus far the routine treatment of cases with a normal anterior segment was discussed. But also in the presence of a pathological anterior segment the four-loop iris clip lens and the two-loop (irido-) capsular lens offer many possibilities for insertion, as is the case after trauma of after previous surgery. This is especially important after trauma where rehabilitation in another way is not adequate, not possible, not wanted, or professionally not allowed. It is impossible to describe the implantation strategy for every possible case, but a few general rules can be given for frequently occurring situations (BINKHORST, 1973).

a. The aphakic eye.

For reason of vitreous problems the intracapsular aphakic eye is a delicate subject for secondary lens implantation and as a rule should be left alone. If an implantation is going to be undertaken, a four loop iris clip lens is inserted in vertical position with a transiridectomy loop suture. Adhesions of the pupillary border to the vitreous face may have to be loosened before implantation.

The extracapsular aphakic eye offers not more risk for secondary im-

115

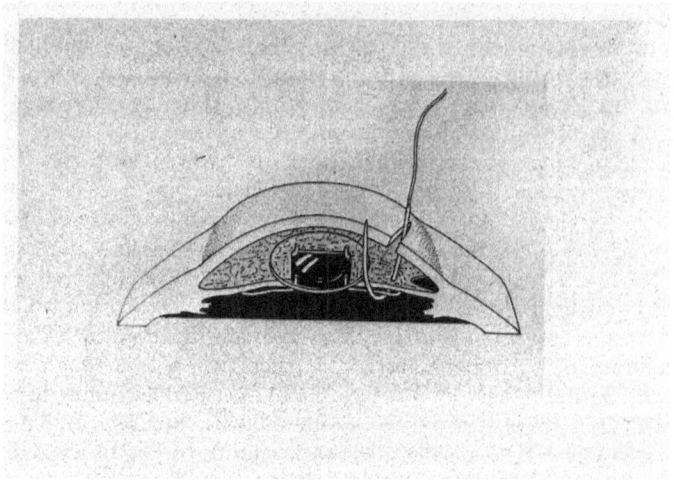

Fig. 26. Transcorneal loop to iris stitch (Binkhorst-Mc Cannell technique).

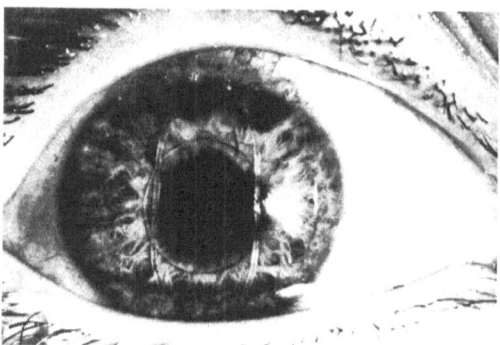

Fig. 27. Extracapsular aphakic eye after implantation of a four-loop iris clip lens, as a secondary procedure. The lens is secured with a transiridectomy loop suture. There were no iris synechiae.

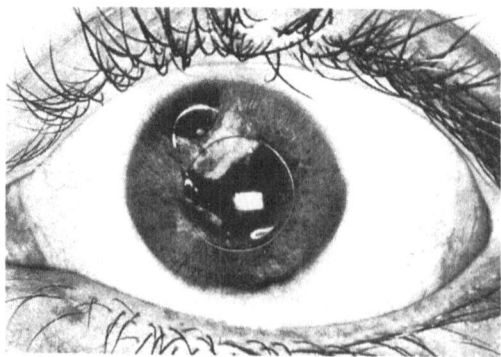

Fig. 28. Two-loop (irido-) capsular lens in a traumatic aphakic eye. The lower loop could be inserted between iris and capsular membrane, but the upper loop had to be inserted behind the capsular membrane through a small capsular membrane incision.

116

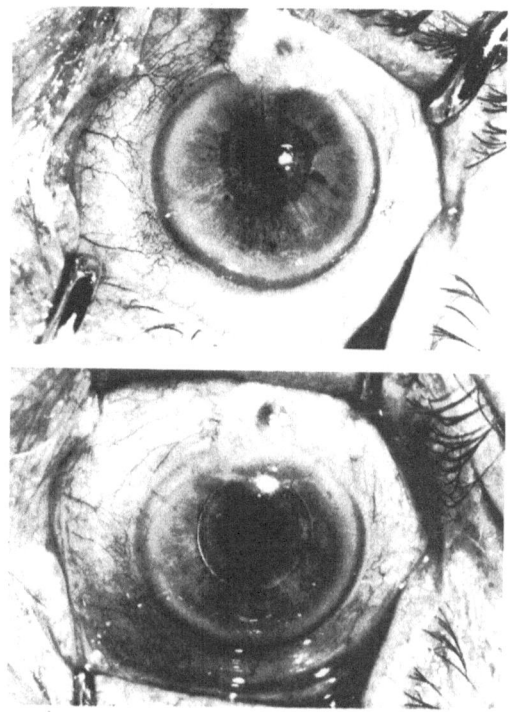

Fig. 29 a. Cataract after previous glaucoma surgery. The pupil is rigid.
b. Same eye with four-loop iris clip lens, inserted through a pre-bleb corneal incision and after performing iridotomy that subsequently was sutured up again.

plantation than does just a second operation. If there are no posterior iris synechiae a four loop lens should be used, secured with a transiridectomy loop suture at 12 o'clock (Fig. 27). It can not be expected that in such a case the presence of the lens will give rise to the formation of adhesions of any kind. If there are irido-capsular adhesions the extent of these is decisive for the strategy to be followed. Sometimes there are two opposite pockets available, at the same time small and big enough to bury the loops of a two-loop lens and keep the lens safely in place. If there are only few synechiae, these should be loosened and the lens loops inserted exactly at these sites in order to have the loops embedded in the synechiae that will be reforming. In case there is a complete seclusion of the pupil, it is sometimes possible to cut them partly so as to form two opposite pockets. If this is not possible the capsular membrane can be incised at the pupillary border and the loops placed underneath the irido-capsular membrane (Fig. 28).

b. The eye after glaucoma surgery

Often there are posterior synechiae of a rigid and narrow pupil. Through a pre-bleb corneal incision and a peripheral coloboma an iridotomy has to be made which after intracapsular cataract extraction and insertion of the lens is closed with two-preplaced perlon sutures (Fig. 29).

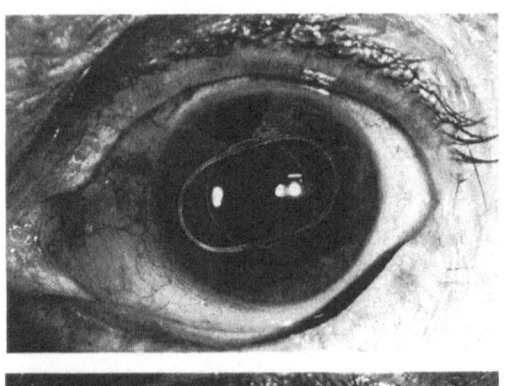

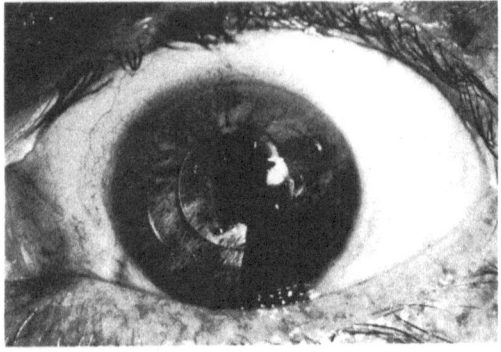

Fig. 30 a. Four-loop iris clip lens inserted into an eye with previous sector iridotomy for acute glaucoma attack. Suturing of the coloboma.
b. Idem into an eye with traumatic sector coloboma of the iris. Perlon bridge between the coloboma pillars.

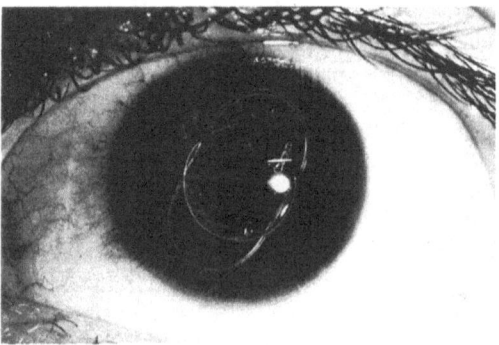

Fig. 31. Contusion 'coloboma' of the temporal-inferior iris sector. Four-loop iris clip lens kept in place by a lens to iris suture in the nasal-superior sector.

c. The eye with iris coloboma

After intracapsular extraction the lens gets easily decentered into the coloboma and thus suturing of the coloboma is necessary. If the defect is wide a perlon bridge between the two ends of the pupillary border will do the same job (Fig. 30). An alternative solution has been to suture the lens

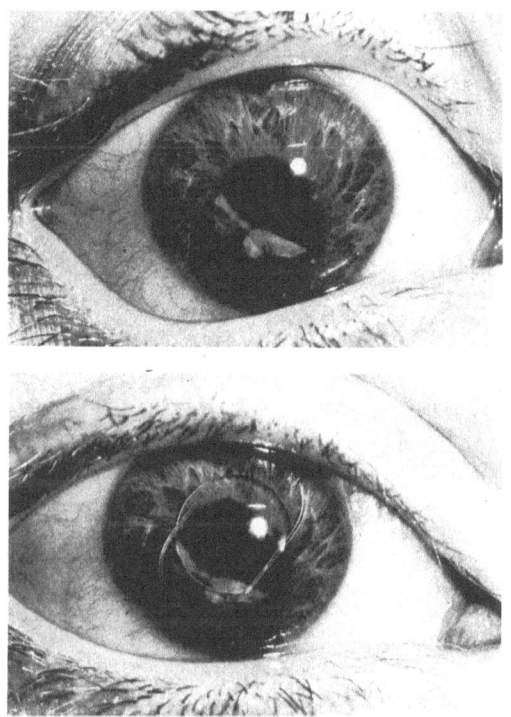

Fig. 32 a. Contusion 'coloboma' of the iris at 6 o'clock. The anterior capsula and some cortex is left in the colobomatous area.
b. Same eye with four-loop lens that is supported by the capsular membrane in the 'coloboma'.

with an anterior loop to the iris in order to prevent displacement (Fig. 31). The favourite procedure to deal with colobomas however is the extra-capsular extraction whilst leaving the anterior capsula untouched in the colobomatous area, where first the anterior capsula and later the capsular membrane gives support for the lens and prevents displacement into the

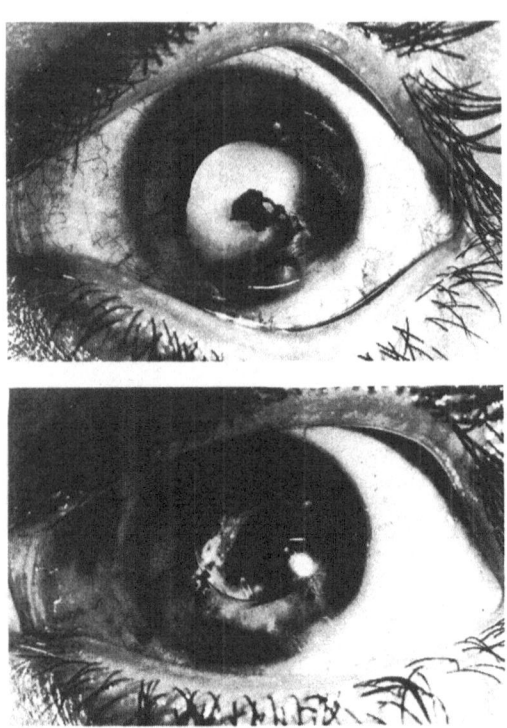

Fig. 33 a. Eye of a 14 year old boy after removal of a big traumatic iris cyst.
b. Same eye after one stage surgery: extracapsular removal of the cataract and implantation of a two-loop lens. Anterior capsule and some cortex are left in the coloboma in order to support the lens.

coloboma (Figs. 32,33). In an already aphakic eye the procedure to be followed is determined by the presence and the extent of irido-capsular adhesions.

120

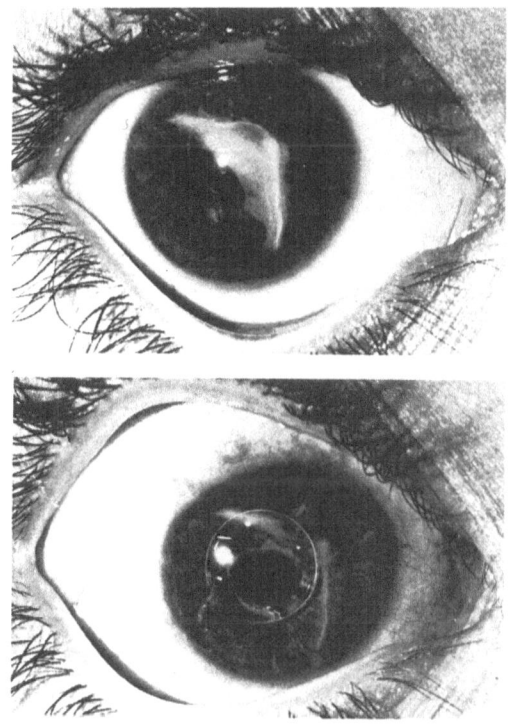

Fig. 34 a. Perforating injury of cornea and crystalline lens. Extensive anterior synechiae.
b. Same eye after dissection of anterior synechiae, extracapsular removal of lens remnants, implantation of a two-loop lens and subsequent excision of part of the capsular
membrane.

d. Anterior synechiae and adhering leucoma.

Anterior synechiae that are not continuous into the chamber angle simply
can be cut whereafter the lens prevents its recurrence (Fig. 34). If however

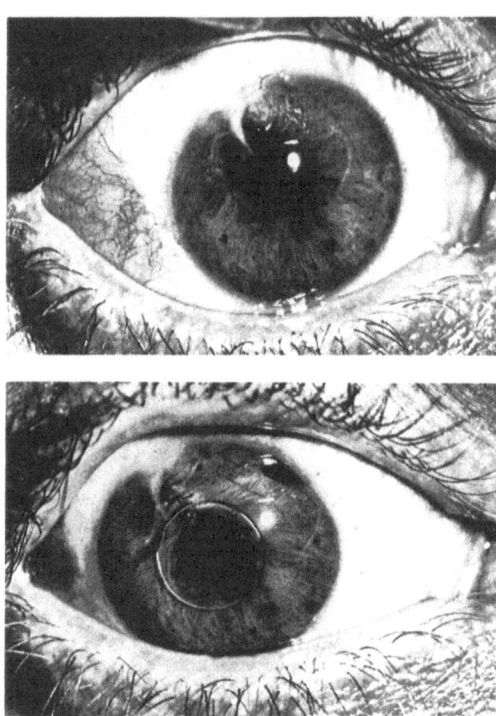

Fig. 35 a. Traumatic aphakic eye with corneal leucoma. Shallow anterior chamber and pupil decentration caused by anterior synechiae of the iris.
b. Same eye with two-loop lens. The chamber is deepened and the lens is centered by performing iridotomies on both sides of the leucoma and subsequent suturing of the leucoma.

continuous into the chamber angle a recurrent adhering processus is likely to flatten the chamber again afterwards. The solution of this problem is to perform iridotomy on both sides of the adhesion and, if necessary, to suture the resulting iris coloboma (Figs. 35, 36).

122

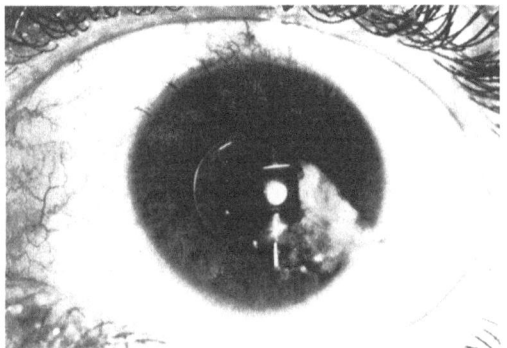

Fig. 36. Traumatic aphakic eye with a corneal leucoma, involving iris and lens membrane. To deepen the anterior chamber, the iris was dissected from the leucoma at 6 o'clock. The lens is supported by the lens membrane.

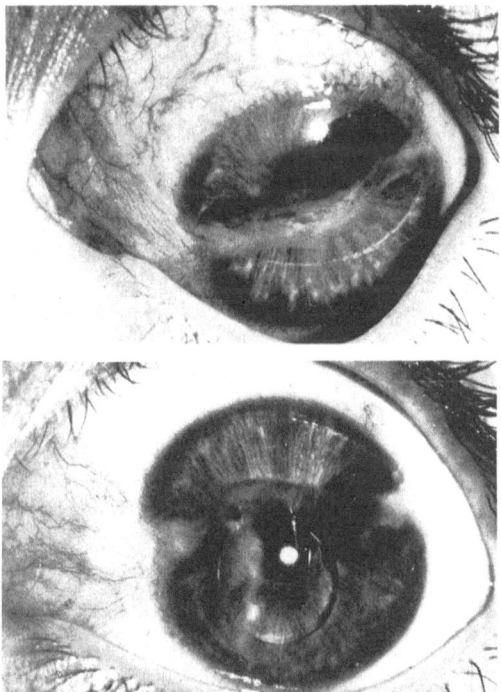

Fig. 37 a. Traumatic aphakia in a four year old girl. Colobomata of the iris. Dense corneal scar occluding the pupillary area.
b. Same eye after one stage surgery; corneal trephining, insertion of a two-loop lens and resuturing of the corneal disk after 90 degree rotation.

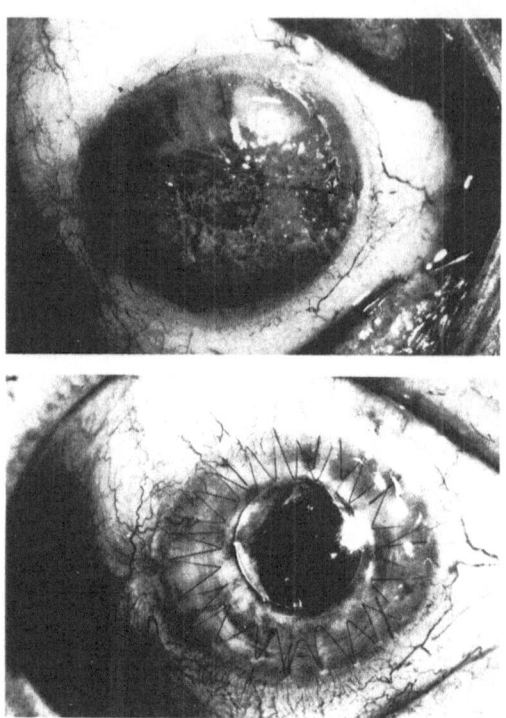

Fig. 38 a. Severe corneal degeneration in a aphakic eye.
b. Same eye after combined implantation of a two-loop lens and keratoplasty.

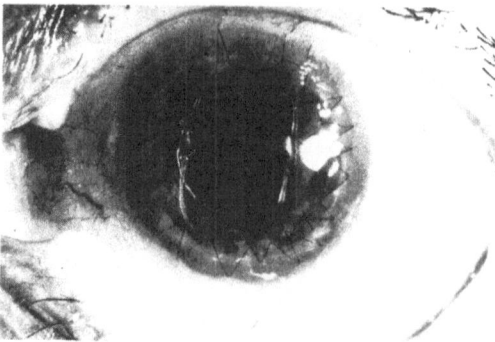

Fig. 39. Combined operation for cataract and Fuchs' corneal dystrophy: intracapsular cataract extraction, implantation of a four-loop lens, secured with transiridectomy loop suture and keratoplasty.

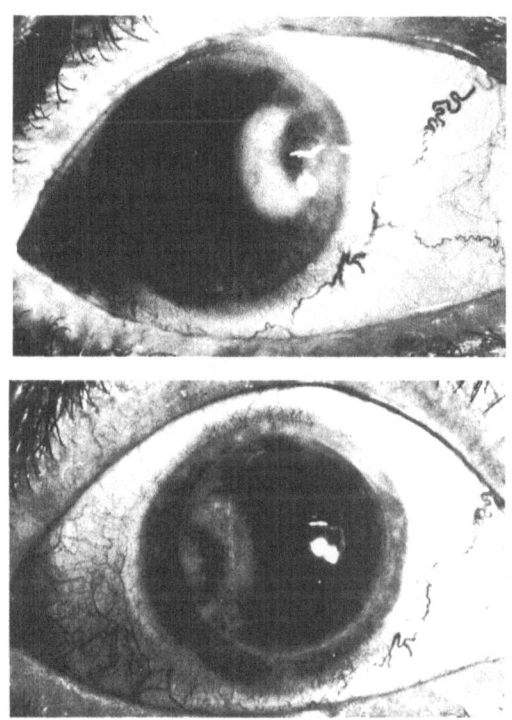

Fig. 40 a. Corneal opacity and cataract.
b. Same eye after combined intracapsular cataract extraction, implantation of a four-looplens, secured with a transiridectomy loop suture, and rotating autokeratoplasty.

e. Cataract and corneal opacity ('combined operation').

Also in these cases combined surgery for cataract, implantation and keratoplasty usually gives very good results (Figs. 37,38,39,40,41).

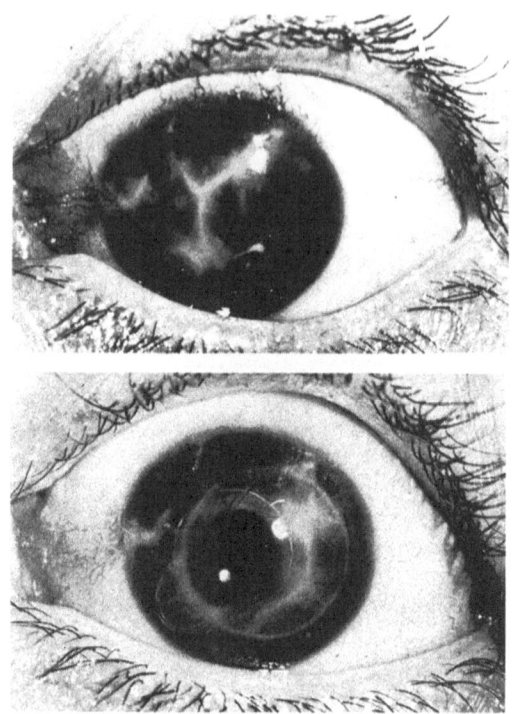

Fig. 41 a. Extensive corneal scarring, aniridia and aphakia after glass injury.
b. Same eye after insertion of a two-loop lens into the capsular membrane and rotating autokeratoplasty. The lens is in inverted position.

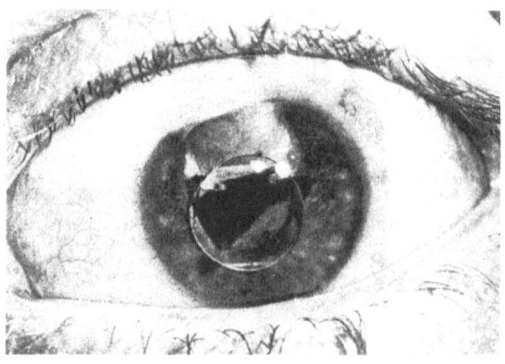

Fig. 42. Traumatic pseudophakic eye after incision of the capsular membrane.

f. Capsular membranes.

If obstructing visual acuity these can be incised, or even excised, preferably after lens implantation, as a secondary procedure (Figs. 42, 43).

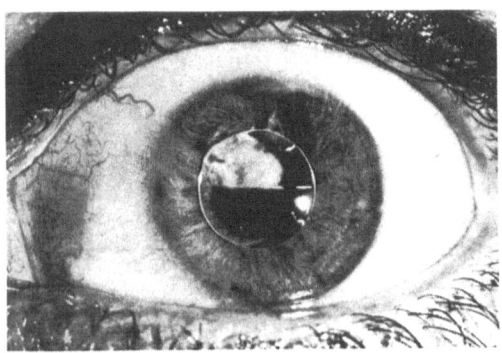

Fig. 43. Traumatic pseudophakic eye after excision of the capsular membrane.

COMMENT AND CONCLUSIONS.

A gross historical survey shows that iris and capsular membrane fixation have rescued intraocular lenses from for ever being forgotten. The author's personal experience of nearly 20 years in more than 1250 implantations of various lens designs, include more than 1150 implantations with iris and capsular support. Implantation has been carried out in many a case of pathological anterior segment.

Very good results were and are obtained with iris support after intracapsular cataract extraction. However capsular fixation after extracapsular cataract extraction offers fixation of higher quality. At the same time extracapsular pseudophakics profit from the advantages they have over intracapsular pseudophakics as to surgical complications and as so the long-term fate of the eye. The extracapsular cataract extraction and implantation of a two--loop (irido-) capsular lens is a method of treatment of senile cataract, that is safe enough to be generalized. An intraocular lens, 'glued' upon the 'dead' capsular membrane, using cortex material as the crystallines own 'glue', approximates the ideal solution of the problem of intraocular lens fixation, viz. stable fixation with minimal tissue contact.

REFERENCES

BARON, A. Tolérance de l'oeil à la matière plastique. Prothèses optiques cornéennes. Prothèses optique cristalliniennes. *Bull.Soc.Ophtal. Paris* 9: *982-988* (1953).

BINKHORST, C.D. Iris supported artificial pseudophakia. A new development in intraocular artificial lens surgery (iris clip lens). *Tr.Ophthal.Soc.U.K.* *79:569-584* (1959).

BINKHORST C.D. The iridocapsular (two-loop) lens and the iris-clip (four-loop) lens in pseudophakia. *Tr.AmAc.Ophthal. and Otolaryng.* *589-617* (Sept-Okt. 1973).

BINKHORST, C.D. & LEONARD, P.A.M. Results in 208 iris clip pseudophakos implantations. *Am.J.Ophthal.* 64: *947-956* (1967).

BINKHORST, C.D., KATS A. & LEONARD, P.A.M. Extracapsular pseudophakia. Results in 100 two-loop iridocapsular lens implantations. *Am.J.Ophthal.* 73: *625-636* (1972).

CHOYCE D.P. Long-term tolerance of Choyce's Mark I and Mark VIII anterior chamber implants. *Proc.Royal Soc.Med.* 63: *310-313* (1970).

EPSTEIN E. Modified Ridley lenses. *Br.J.Ophthal.* 43: *29-33* (1959).

FEDOROV, S.N. Personal communication.

FEDOROV, S.N.: cited by BINKHORST C.D. in: Lens implants (pseudophakoi) classified according to method of fixation. *Br.J.Ophthal.* 51: *772-774* (1967).

LEONARD P.A.M. Personal communication.

LURIE L. Personal communication.

MANSCHOT W.A. Histopathology of eyes containing Binkhorst lenses. *Am.J.Ophthal.* In press.

NORDLOHNE M.E. Dislocation and endothelial corneal dystrophy (ECD) in patients fitted with Binkhorst lens implants (1958-1972), this volume: *15-22.*

RIDLEY, H. Intraocular acrylic lenses. *Tr.Ophthal.Soc.U.K.* 71: *617-621* (1951).

RIDLEY, H. Late surgical results of use of the intraocular acrylic lens. *J.Int.Coll.Surg.* 26: *335-341* (1956).

SCHILLINGER, R.J. SHEARER, R.V. & LEVY, O.R. Animal experiments with a new type of intraocular acrylic lens. *Arch.Ophthal.* 59: *423-434* (1958).

STRAMPELLI B. Sopportabilità di lenti acriliche in camera anteriore nella afachia e nei viz di refrazione. *An Ottal.* 80: *75-82* (1954).

WORST, J.G.F. L'implantation d'un cristallin artificiel (iris clip lens de Binkhorst). *Bull.MemSoc.Fr.Ophtal.* *84-547* (1971).

WORST, J.G.F., Ned. Oogheelk. Gezelschap, Rotterdam (Dec. 1973).

WORST, J.G.F., LUDWIG H.H.H. & MASSARO, R.G. Binkhorst's artificial lens. Proc. XXI International Congress of Ophthal. Excerpta Medica International Congress Series no. 222, pp. 776-780.

HISTOPATHOLOGY OF EYES CONTAINING
BINKHORST LENSES

W.A. MANSCHOT

(Rotterdam)

ABSTRACT

Of 2,724 eyes in which a Binkhorst lens was implanted before 1972, only one eye, containing an iridocapsular lens, had to be enucleated because of a postoperative complication. This eye and postmortem eyes from this series, and one more eye operated on at a later date were studied histopathologically. Corneal dystrophy and glaucoma were in no case the reason for enucleation. Epithelial downgrowth was not observed. Two postmortem eyes from one patient showed marked infiltration by lymphocytes and proliferation of stromal cells in the central superficial part of the iris stroma. A constant finding in all eyes containing an iris clip lens was multiple pressure atrophy of the pupillary border with interruption of the sphincter muscle. This atrophy appeared due to pressure exerted by the attachments of the posterior wire loops; it appeared less severe in eyes containing iridocapsular lenses. No macular edema or cystic macular degeneration was observed.

The whole article has been published in: *Amer.J,Ophthal.* 1974, Vol. 77.

OOSTERHUIS: First of all we start with the indications for performing implant surgery. We heard just now from BINKHORST about the cases of injuries and he showed us quite a lot of pictures about that and told us which is a very strong indication. I want to ask him, because he has the most experience of the panel of implant surgery in children, what is his opinion on implant surgery in congenital cataract? At what age it has to be done in the first place?

BINKHORST: Congenital cataract surgery is surgery in a normal segment, so it should not offer too many difficulties, but you must realise that the infant eye offers difficulties of its own, and everyone of you knows that. I do not think it is right to make an incision in an infant eye of more than one or two millimeters and the consequence of this is that in very young eyes now to-day I refuse to do implants. I must confess that I have done it. The earliest age was 8 months. But to-day I refuse to do that under the age of, let us say 2 years. But then you wonder what indications are left. Now it is not the unilateral congenital cataract, because from the functional point of view, that is much too late. It may be questioned if you have better results with earlier operation, personally I do not think so. What is left is the subtotal cataract, for instance a zonular cataract. They usually turn out to have insufficient vision at the age of 3,4,5,6 even, and when vision is insufficient something has to be done. Now I think implant surgery in this field is of great advantage because when we operate the eye with the lowest visual acuity and leave the other eye untouched, we have a child that has been operated on one eye only. It has to face perhaps complications in his later life, but only in one eye. The alternative would have been to operate both eyes to save the binocular vision that often is present in these infants.
So, summarizing, I would say: The unilateral cataract should be left untouched, and the bilateral partial cataract is a good indication, but only at the age of 4, 5 years.

OOSTERHUIS: Thank you. Dr. WORST, your comment on that. You have experience at very young age.

WORST: Yes, I have done traumatic cases and I had to design a special completely new technique for insertion because

131

the regular technique failed. It would go too far which technique this is, but it works with two small incisions and a traction suture and a keratome which is loaded with an injection canule to keep the anterior chamber filled; it is a whole factory to get it in and it worked technically speaking, though the functional results were very difficult to maintain because of the amblyopia treatment. I am speaking about extremely difficult traumatic cases, however, I have no experience in congenital cases, but I would like to mention that technically it is possible using a special traction suture technique.

OOSTERHUIS: Thank you. Dr. JAFFE do you have experience with very young children?

JAFFE: I personally feel that at this stage of my own development and at this stage of the development of intraocular lenses the insertion of intraocular lenses into eyes with congenital cataract is really a hazardous experience. I think there are very few of us who could sit here to-day and say that this eye will tolerate such a lens for the rest of the lifetime of that eye, and I personally would shy away from this. What the experience that we are now beginning to accumulate is, as mentioned by Dr. BINKHORST is a very simple aspiration of a congenital cataract and then the use of a Griffin lens, a soft lens of the Griffin variety. And this is the experience that we are beginning to accumulate. These lenses can be left on the eye for many months at a time and with intelligent parents they can just be taken off on rare occasions for cleaning to avoid infection. But I think we are really embarking on something a little dangerous to put something inside these very young eyes when we can keep something on the outside of the eye which can do almost as well. Unfortunately it is very difficult to strive for a perfection in these eyes and we should just do the best we can to prevent amblyopia. So my feeling at the current time is what we are doing is the use of a Griffin soft lens.

OOSTERHUIS: Thank you very much Dr. JAFFE. Dr. BINKHORST will you please comment on this?

BINKHORST: I suppose that Dr. JAFFE spoke about bilateral operation in congenital cataract or a unilateral operation?

JAFFE: I am talking specifically about both. In the first place with the unilateral cataract, I am quite in agreement with you, that almost no matter what you do with the unilateral congenital cataract your results will not be very exceptional. You than made the distinction between the so-called developmental cataract, or let us say congenital cataract and a zonular cataract. The zonular cataract, we all agree, is much easier to treat and I think I would still like to go on the side of conservatism and I would still like to satisfy myself because I had cases such as this where dilation of the pupil gives adequate functional results to vision 20/60 to 20/70, and it is in my opinion that a 20/60 or 20/70 eye that can still perform accommodation is a better eye than an aphakic eye. If dilation improves the vision to a satisfactorily level, in the United States to attent the regular school you need 20/70 vision in the better eye, and if I can accomplish this I would much rather perform an optical iridectomy.

OOSTERHUIS: Thanks. Now we will proceed to the indications for surgery in the adults. We all know that there are many different opinions. Not only opinions, but some people say: Well, I am only doing it at the age of 70 or more; others say: Well, I do it in very many cases, and once I heard Jan WORST say to me: Patients must have very strong contra-indications not to get an implant lens, and I very much want to hear what are these contra-indications and why?

WORST: Contra-indication number one is the condition of the eye that is on the surgical table. This is often forgotten: that it must be possible to insert the lens, and any time one fears that it is technically impossible to perform the operation that is contra-indication number one. Do not try to go on, even when someone watches, or when the patient has asked for a lens implant. The patient has to be informed in this matter that he may receive an implant if things are favourable.
Second absolute contra-indication is diabetes, a manifest diabetes in the relatively young.
Third contra-indication is dystrophies, corneal dystrophy of any kind.
Fourth contra-indication is, well, in my opinion I do not dare to touch the young, very young children when they have congenital cataract. I had rather refer them to someone with more experience in this field.
Glaucoma and cataract used to be a contra-indication and it is not any more. Cataract and glaucoma, I mean the combination of the disease and cataract is not a contra-indication anymore, but I used to call it for myself an absolute contra-indication. It has become relative.
Myopia over minus 10 diopters.
Previous detachment surgery.
Aniseikonia problems which I cannot solve because I have

problems in calculating and have fears that I may cause an aniseikonia, in which case the patient is referred to a special clinic where calculations are done in advance.

And that is about all, but in practice it results in the situation that roughly 90-95% of the cataract patients of the simple senile cataract receive an intraocular lens in my area.

There must be more contra-indications, but for the moment I cannot think of more.

A voice: An unsteady marriage?

WORST: Yes. Psychological. That is a whole story which I did not go into, the whole range of: what is the person, what does he want, what is the binocular function, does he need it.

OOSTERHUIS: Thank you. You have named different contra-indications which in themselves are worthwhile to have discussion on it, but I want to do it on only one thing and that is the corneal dystrophy. You say that this is a contra-indication for an implant and I think BINKHORST has a different opinion about it.

BINKHORST: Yes, I think the contrary, because if you operate an ordinary cataract in a dystrophic cornea that is reasonably clear, you certainly will end up with a much more opaque cornea than you started with. Corneal dystrophies, senile corneal dystrophy, is a progressive disease and sooner or later you are forced to do a keratoplasty and you are in a much better position to do a keratoplasty in an eye with an implant lens than in an aphakic eye, and for that reason I should think a corneal dystrophy is an urgent indication for an implant lens.

WORST: I know, but the waiting list for corneal transplant in my area is 2-3 years. Many times decisions of this kind are determined by the local situation. Another point I forgot to mention is absence of proper assistance and absence of the right anesthesist. That is another technical contra-indication which is very important to realise, if one is forced to do it on local anesthesia it is quite possible that the situation is too difficult.

OOSTERHUIS: Professor DRAEGER, will you comment on this?

DRAEGER: Besides the problem Dr. WORST has mentioned I personally would completely agree with Dr. BINKHORST. We all know that after normal cataract extraction a severe Fuchs dystrophy gets worse, so why not try to combine?

We have not the experience Dr. BINKHORST has and not so many impressing cases, but a small number of combined operations proved his opinion and so we are in agreement not to believe Fuchs dystrophy an absolute contraindication. You have to deal with the dystrophy, but you can.

OOSTERHUIS: Thank you very much. Now I want to hear the comment of Dr. JAFFE.

JAFFE: The big problem is the decision about the cornea. To make a distinction between an advanced case of so-called cornea guttata and the kind that we call Fuchs dystrophy on a clinical basis is extremely difficult. I have never been successful in making this determination. If you have a history of decompensation with epithelial oedema it makes it very simple for you. Unfortunately, many of these clear spontaneously and the ophthalmic surgeon never gets an oppertunity to see these patients during stages of decompensation. Only a history of an occasional 'I feel something in my. eye' type of thing. So it becomes very difficult and much to one's chagrin one operates on an eye with what looks like guttata and is chagrined to see that within a short period postoperatively the patient has a full-blown corneal dystrophy. Now, as I stated earlier to-day, I find that these are very excellent prognostic eyes to do surgery on. If I have a patient, whom I have observed with Fuchs dystrophy, who also has a dense cataract, in whom I feel an intraocular lens is indicated, I will do all three procedures together. But I still must say that I like to proceed on the conservative side, and whenever there is a complicating factor, such as those mentioned by Dr. WORST, I would like to shy away from intraocular lenses. Any complicating factor, anything new for the eye tends to shy me away. In other words: Why add another problem to an operation which, at least in mỳ hands, has caused more complications than routine cataract surgery. And that is my current feeling. When many people visit us from other cities in the United States, I tell them, that if I hear that they are doing more than 10 to 15% of their extractions with implants, I will feel that they got nothing out of their instruction at our institution. That we preach conservatism, that we teach that these things should be done in a minimum of cases. Now we are not all BINKHORST and WORST and we do not have the background and experience, but in the United States to-day I every now and then will get a report 'that so-and-so left your institution and is now doing 95% intraocular lenses'. But it is only because he is so spastic, and so young, and so immature, that he is anxious to build up a series within a very brief period of time to have more than all his colleagues in his city. So usually what we do is to call a person like that and say: Where did you learn to do so many?, and hope to slow them down. Now this is not a reflection on the work that I have seen presented here by Dr. BINKHORST to-day, because after spending time with him I realise, and after looking at the cases, that these are splendid-looking eyes, and I probably will have to rearrange my thinking in the next few years, but it will only be done on the basis of my own personal experience.

OOSTERHUIS: Thank you very much. Dr. LEEMAN, do you have an experience with this combination of dystrophy and cataract?

LEEMAN: No, I already said so, but I think I agree with Dr. BINK-HORST and Dr. JAFFE that you should do it in combination, because I think otherwise it will end up as a dystrophic eye anyway.

OOSTERHUIS: Yes, thank you. Well, I agree with that and I think that perhaps in case the facilities for Dr. WORST should be such that he would not have a waiting list of several years or a proper assistant to help him perhaps he would revise his opinion.

WORST: I have one technical remark about the diagnosis. The best way to see it is just with the operating microscope and the anterior chamber filled with air. It is remarkable how clearly then suddenly the dystrophy shows up.

JAFFE: But is not that the way guttata looks also? When you do the same thing it looks the same to me.

BINKHORST: May I make one remark. It should not be misunderstood that I advise a combined operation, keratoplasty and cataract and implantation, in every case of guttata, cornea guttata. For me the indication for a combined operation is really a stromal oedema, even if it is very small.

OOSTERHUIS: Thank you. I think we leave this topic and we go on with the next. We have heard about the contra-indications and now I want to hear from Dr. BINKHORST what he thinks to be very strong indications in the adult.

BINKHORST: Once, and I have said that before the Dutch Ophthalmological Society once, I thought that an eye that had been operated for glaucoma should have an implant after cataract removal, and that opinion was based on the experiences, I think of MAUMENEE, who reviewed hundreds of glaucoma operated eyes that were made aphakic and in which he in 60% found a decompensation of the intraocular pressure. So this for me is not an absolute, but it is a heavily weighing indication in an adult.

Other strong indications, there are no absolute indications of course, but a strong indication is the professional indication. I remember, and Professor TEN DOESSCHATE will remember, that he sent me a jet pilot that he had devaluated for his profession, and that man had a 0.6 vision in his cataractous eye and a normal in the other eye. Now usually I do not operate on an eye with 0.6 vision, but it was a challenge and the man begged me for that, and I did it and, if you go to New York, he will probably fly you back to New York!

OOSTERHUIS: May I ask from the panel: Are there any other suggestions for very strong indications? Because ophthalmologists sitting here want to know. They want to do it themselves and they want to know the strong indications.

JAFFE: If we are talking about senile cataracts, for me, as I mentioned earlier, a very excellent indication is that patient with a mature cataract in one eye and relatively usable , but not very good vision in the second eye, like 20/50, 20/60 or 20/70, particularly if that eye performs poorly in the sun and he has difficulty in reading. And if the patient is very elderly, like over 75 for example, I will consider this a very strong indication, because in that way I need do only one operation on this person for usually the rest of his lifetime.

And the other strong indication I mentioned earlier today, and I would hope that others here would be in to examine this position, to see if it is as correct as we say it is, is the use of lens implants in patients with known disciform macular degeneration. I really consider this to be one of the strongest indications in those who have this degeneration, who then subsequently develop a disabling cataract which cuts their vision from the usual 24/100 down to perhaps hand motion or light perception. These are some of the most grateful patients with a retention of their peripheral field. These are two of the most urgent indications for me.

OOSTERHUIS: Thank you very much. Professor DRAEGER also wants to comment on this.

DRAEGER: One very strong indication was not yet mentioned. I had a

137

patient last week with a really urgent indication, a lady of early 60, with a strictly unilateral cataract. I did BINK-HORST implant four years ago and now she had a mature cataract on the other eye. This is a strong indication too.

OOSTERHUIS: Now please hear Dr. BINKHORST.

BINKHORST: There may be a patient that has been operated and has been made aphakic and tells you that she cannot tolerate the contact lens and that she is going to commit suicide if you do not implant the other eye. It has happened to me.

JAFFE: May I ask for my own education: What is the experience with an implant in one eye and a contact lens in the other eye? I got the impression to-day that you almost have to do the implant in the second eye. Our experience in Miami has been, that these patients function extremely well and it is less hazardous to them if you put an implant in just one eye, and do a routine cataract extraction with a contact lens in the opposite eye. With the implant eye they see well enough to manage the contact lens on their finger. And there is no such thing to-day as not being able to tolerate a contact lens: if not a hard lens it will be a soft lens with even correction of residual refractive error if there is too much astigmatism. But I am really not so overly impressed by the importance in these people of what we are talking about with a very sophisticated form of binocular vision. I think most patients perform very well, particularly the elderly patients, with a more rudimentary form of binocular vision, particularly a peripheral type of fusion. And at least in our community I would like to err on that side and not expose the patient to two intraocular lenses. I have done bilateral implants, but I would prefer to do it the other way and I would like to know of those who have more experience: What is so bad about an implant in one eye and a contact lens in the other eye?

OOSTERHUIS: May I ask another question: What is so bad about having two implants?

JAFFE: It is very difficult for me to answer such a question. I must just tell you that it is my personal nature and the nature of those around me, who feel that if something goes wrong with the implant in that eye, for example perhaps cystoid macular oedema, which is a big problem, and if it is persistent in one eye, in our experience this becomes a grave problem. And now you have a patient with two implants in the eye and now two cystoid macular oedemas and two 20/400 eyes. And sometimes, if you take these lenses out the cystoid macular oedema does not improve. So I only mention this as one possible complication. There might be others, that I am not even aware of, but at any rate it seems to me to be safer to put only one implant in than to put in two. That is almost irreligious to say, perhaps, here, but that is the way I feel about it.

OOSTERHUIS: But I think this needs some comment, some further comment of the panel and I start with Dr. BINKHORST.

BINKHORST: Now I want just to bring you back to NORMAN JAFFE, We should distinguish between the type of aphakia and sort of aphakia. Either we are dealing with intracapsular or extracapsular eyes. Especially as regards the occurrence of cystoid macular oedema.

JAFFE: Well, the cystoid macular oedema that I see in the normal intracapsular lens extraction, I think I have spoken about this in Amsterdam, in Rotterdam and in Nijmegen, and I feel that almost 100% of intracapsular lens extractions have during their postoperative history at some time leakage of fluorescein into the macula and therefore Irvine Gass syndrome. But in the overwhelming majority of these, these are transient. Persistent cystoid macular oedema is probably not found in more than 1,2% of intracapsular lens extractions without an implant. And I just would not accept any other figures about implant cystoid macular oedema unless somebody actually has the facts and the numbers, and the statistics, and the proof, to tell me that the numbers are the same in that condition.

WORST. You are quoting very high figures, Norman, and it is quite possible that it is typical of your country.

JAFFE: No. you misunderstood. The high figures that I have described first were in those without implants. You understood that Jan, that I believe that 100% of normal intracapsular lens extractions without pseudophakos have some type of macular oedema, not some type of cystoid macular oedema. Incompetent intraretinal capillaries with an oedema in the outer plexiform layer of Henle that acts like a sponge and all the fluid collects in it, but in most instances this disappears.

OOSTERHUIS: Professor DRAEGER.

DRAEGER: I should like to put Dr. JAFFE's question concerning the unilateral operation the other side. Dr. BINKHORST, would you go on with implanting a lens in a successfully operated case being happy with a contact lens on the first eye?

BINKHORST: No.

OOSTERHUIS: May I ask WORST, you have done an implant lens and the patient has a normal vision a long time, and well, there has to be made a decision about the second eye. Are you going to operate on the second eye?

WORST: I am faced frequently with the following situation: The patient cannot tolerate the contact lens and develops a cataract in the other eye. This patient will receive an artificial lens and of then he would come back and pressurize me to start implanting on the other eye, which I usually refuse and refuse again. But some of them become so obnoxious and are so depressed about it, that in a few instances I have done a secondary implantation in an already successfully operated aphakic eye. Some of them have come out favourably and in some I have regretted it.

DRAEGER: No, not this way, no personal experience.

OOSTERHUIS: And Dr. LEEMAN?

LEEMAN: I think it depends on the age of the patient. When the patient has an implant in one eye and everything is allright and he is very old, I think you are allowed to do the other eye, but when he is younger, especially when he is 50 or younger, you should not do it.

OOSTERHUIS: Now, we are now making the problem more simple and we leave out the second eye and take only the patients having one eye, one useful eye, the monocular patients. I want to hear in that case, what would you do, is this a contra-indication, Jan, I did not hear that from you in your list of contra-indications.

WORST: I remember exactly the three cases. Monocular cases where I have implanted, I can call them in, they are doing very well, I have done it, I have taken all the possible precautions I could take, I have not regretted it, my series contains I think three. One of them is my neighbour, it is a woman to whom I lived nextdoor, and I could see her for several years daily. If it is true that lens implantation is a correct procedure I cannot see why it could not be applied to a unilateral case. There is always the inference that we are doing something potentially risky. I agree to

140

disincline in this respect.

OOSTERHUIS: Is there anyone on the panel who did also operate on monocular cases?

BINKHORST: I did it once in an eye that had been operated for glaucoma, but I did it for a special purpose. You must not forget that when a one-eyed patient comes to you he probably has already been operated on his other eye and lost that eye for some reason or the other, for an iritis, uveitis, glaucoma and so on. You should be very suspicious for the second eye, for the oculus ultimus.

WORST: Yes Kees, that is true, but I always ask carefully what was the reason of the loss of the first eye, and that could be that it was just a surgical error committed somewhere else, and I am then forewarned not to repeat that.

OOSTERHUIS: Norman JAFFE wants to comment.

JAFFE: I really could not care if the surgical error was elsewhere or whereever it was. Personally in your series of three, Jan, and I do not mean to needle you, but we might as well have a little fun here, because if we are all going to agree then everybody will go to sleep. So therefore I would like to say that if you have a series of three and your fourth is a disaster, your statistics have changed very drastically! I would also like to state that, personally, I could never, never consider, if this were my eye, even letting Dr. BINKHORST put a lens, if that were my only eye. I know exactly the kind of surgery that I would like to-day done on my only eye, and for sure, it would nòt be with an intraocular lens inside of it. And again, I apologize for saying that here in The Netherlands, but that is the way it is.

Applause.

OOSTERHUIS: Now the next question: We already heard about the use and the possibilities of the soft lens. And one of the questions I had myself is: If you think that in the future, the soft lenses will be tolerated better than they are now, this may cause a change in the indications for performing implant lenses.

JAFFE: We have a, I would say, pretty fair experience now with soft lenses and I would say that the experience has been relatively happy. I think the big problem with the soft lens, and I know all of those of you who have used it know that this is a problem, is the residual astigmatism of your cataract surgery. Now again, those of you who heard me speak on the control of astigmatism know that we are spending a great deal of time on this and we now can almost with a routine incision as large as 160° control and reduce our astigmatism from preoperative astigmatism levels practically down to zero with trigonometric calculations. It is not difficult to do, as those of you who did not fall asleep in Amsterdam, Rotterdam, etc. found out. However, the experiences that we are having with soft lenses now is really excellent. The Bausch and Lomb soft lens is a problem. It is too fragile, it turns yellow, it becomes opaque and it still is a problem, even though we have approved it with the Food and Drug Administration. However, the Griffin lens, which we have been using now, has been a very happy experience and we have a group of patients now, on whom we are leaving this Griffin lens in place. I have one lady now, a young lady who had cataract surgery, on whom I have a Griffin lens for 17 months and the lens has not been removed for one minute! So therefore it may change our thinking, it is possible, and we should have open minds on this subject. When technology improves it may actually drive the intraocular lens right out of the ball park and we must be ready for these things. And I would be the first one to be happy with keeping my correction on the outside of the eye rather than the inside of the eye in spite of the excellent results that have been obtained. But I think we must wait now to see what is going to happen. I can tell you that the next lens coming along which Dow Corning is working with the silicone lens, which is a semi-soft lens. One of the problems at this particular time is that of withholding approval with the Food and Drug Administration in the United States. For when this lens becomes popular you will be able to correct astigmatism with it, and you will be able to do more things with the eye that currently we cannot do to-day. So I think we must all be ready for technology to change the things that we do. And I cannot believe that anything we are discussing to-day is here forever. I believe that much of what we are writing is obsolete and anybody like myself who has written a book knows that the day your book appears in print it is obsolete. So we are all going to be obsolete and we are all going to have obsolescent techniques, so we must be prepared for these changes.

OOSTERHUIS: Thank you very much. I think we ask Professor DRAE-GER's comment about it.

DRAEGER: There certainly will be a progress in soft or semi-soft lenses technology. We have a semi-soft lens under trial which is a German production and is very promising and I agree with Dr. JAFFE that this will solve many problems. But there will be a group of contra-indications completely independent from this optical point of view. There are some people which are not able even to handle long wearable lenses as also are very young children with poor care, and not very young children with poor care. Some unilateral cases where we even in the future probably will have to rely on intraocular lenses, even if technology makes progress. This is my opinion about this problem.

OOSTERHUIS: Thank you, I think that we will now leave the subject of the indications despite the fact that there are many more problems and interesting facts which we could discuss. I think we should now proceed about several problems in the technique. And the first thing is that you all have seen the table of Dr. BINKHORST in which the number of cases in which he did an extracapsular extraction increased very rapidly in the course of the last years. My first question is for Dr. BINKHORST, if he thinks that in most of the cases the extracapsular extraction will be the choice in the future.

BINKHORST: Certainly I do. The reason that the increase of the frequency of extracapsular operation was so fast the later years is because I wanted to build up a large series of extracapsulars, planned extracapsulars, as soon as possible. So it is not a natural development, because I thought the intracapsular extraction is so bad. But I realise more and more that the intracapsular extraction giving late complications, giving complications at surgery, is not the basic technique, not the technique of choice for implantation for everyone. And because everyone wants to do implantations, at least it seems so, I jumped upon this extracapsular technique to try if this would be a method to generalize and I think this is a method to generalize much better and with less risk than the intracapsular extraction. Now I am speaking about the surgery itself, but also I feel and not only feel but I am pretty sure that the late complications after extracapsular extractions are less than after intracapsular extractions. And that may be true for detachments, that is certainly true for cystoid macular oedema. So the answer to the question for my part is: Yes, I think that the extracapsular extraction is the future. And you know it all, because I have said that before for the Dutch Ophthalmological Society, and especially with the newer techniques that are developing in the United States I think that this holds even more true.

OOSTERHUIS: Thank you. You did not mention it specifically, but also the corneal dystrophy is a much lower percentage in the extracapsular extraction.

BINKHORST: I forgot that. In our 420 cases of extracapsular extraction we have only one case of corneal dystrophy. That was in a heavy traumatized eye and already the injury itself and the repeated surgery in this eye could have provoked it.

OOSTERHUIS: You are being too modest.

JAFFE: Can I ask a question on that to Dr. BINKHORST. Your follow-up period at the moment on extracapsular extractions is relatively short compared to your exceptionally long follow-up on intracapsular surgery. I also recall your recording at one time in the American Journal of Ophthalmology in other areas zero % corneal dystrophy, which later in 1973 became 3% corneal dystrophy. Is it possible that with the increase in time you might change your ideas about these statistics as you did with intracapsular cataract extraction, because I would like to just criticize in a sense and say that you still do not have the statistics available and you cannot compare them yet with the other because your follow-up period, I believe, is too short.

BINKHORST: That is completely right. The follow-up is much shorter, although it is 4 years, but I agree that in the beginning we had our corneal dystrophies only after 5 to 6 years. I agree with that. There is one point: There is less reason for corneal dystrophy, at least for contact dystrophy, with a lens with two loops.

JAFFE: I believe that Dr. BINKHORST made a very important point when he spoke about phako-emulsification. To those of you who have witnessed the great obstruction to the development of intracapsular lenses, you can only imagine in the United States the great resistance to Dr. KELMAN, when he first presented phako-emulsification. Richard KRATZ was here in this country and was with us with Dr. BINKHORST the other day, and he is probably one of the foremost surgeons for phako-emulsification. And he assures us that he can really clean that posterior capsule and he can give a very uniform 360° type of cortical capsular material present at the equator, so that it will be easier to fix these lenses. And I think that Dr.

BINKHORST feels also that this might be the future and it certainly seems to be to me logical to assume that this will be the future of implant surgery.

OOSTERHUIS: Thank you. I have one remark and that is: Dr. BINKHORST told us that the follow-up period of iridocapsular lenses is about 4 years.

BINKHORST: No it is longer, but the senile cases is about 4, 5 years.

OOSTERHUIS: Yes, but NORDLOHNE told us to-day that the average time for developing corneal dystrophy is about 3 years. So I think that in your series of 4 years and longer, at least in part of the patients epithelial keratopathy should have developed and, well, the ultimate result is not known, but I think that with what you have told us you are slightly too modest and it seems to me not strictly proven but it seems relatively favourable, even very favourable.

BINKHORST: When I reported a zero % of corneal dystrophy after intracapsular extraction I had seen corneas that were a little bit thicker than normal, but they were still completely clear. So later in these cases corneal dystrophy appeared, bullous keratopathy appeared, and I have not seen these unhealthy corneas, and I would like to mention them unhealthy because they are a little bit thicker in extracapsular extractions. We have the tools to measure the corneal thickness and if we have the manpower we are eager to measure corneal thicknesses. I think that is a very good research project.

OOSTERHUIS: Thank you.

WORST: There is some confusion in my mind now and maybe you can clear it up. It is a matter of methodical approach. BINKHORST has shown that the extracapsular technique has a greater stability of the lens and at the same time we know that the instability of the lens is the cause of maybe 90 or more percent of the dystrophies. Is it not correct to conclude from this experience already that it must be right. We talk too much statistics at these times and this takes away the purely logical thinking, clinical logical thinking, which should have a place as well.

OOSTERHUIS: May I ask Professor DRAEGER if he is doing extracapsular extractions as a rule?

DRAEGER: Before coming to Utrecht yesterday I had not the slightest idea to change my intracapsular approach. We have very favourable results and really no problems. So I just start to think about the idea of doing it extracapsularly. But there is one objection to Dr. BINKHORST's idea to generalize this technique by doing it extracapsularly: There is no general knowledge in most eye departments since 50 years or even more to do extracapsular extraction properly. So this is a very awkward idea now to go back with our technique and we do not train our residents this way. Nobody has personal experience in extracapsular extraction and so this is a long and difficult way too to change the whole technique.

OOSTERHUIS: Perhaps you have some emeritus professors which you can ask to give you advice. Now I want to ask Dr. LEEMAN as one of the Dutch ophthalmologists what he is doing.

LEEMAN: In traumatic and unilateral cataracts in patients under the age of 45 I usualy do an extracapsular lensextraction preceding implantation of an artificial lens.
Most of these eyes do well but sometimes I am troubled by the problems arising from the extracapsular technics. At times I leave too much lens-material in the eye, that apart from a delayed restoration of vision sometimes is seen to cause decentration of the lens. In other cases too little lens-material is left causing a poor fixation of the pseudophakoi.
For these reasons I cannot be as enthousiastic as Dr. BINKHORST to advocate the extracapsular extraction in all cases of implant surgery.

OOSTERHUIS: Well, I should say: pay Dr. BINKHORST a visit at his clinic. It might help because from what he showed in his pictures there is scarcely any after-cataract. Now one interesting thing is that we heard to-day Professor DRAEGER tell us that only extraordinary good surgeons do not need an operating microscope. So in case you did not know already, BINKHORST and WORST are very good surgeons, because they do not use a microscope. This is a very interesting fact. I think we need not discuss this, because just look at the results. I only want to put one question: Is it not wise that the younger generation starting with implant surgery should first know very well how to use the operative microscope? But I do not want to put this question to Professor DRAEGER because then I know beforehand what he will say. I will ask this question to Dr. BINKHORST who did most of the implant surgery, but never used the operating microscope, only once I believe, last year in Amsterdam at the television show.

BINKHORST: I did not use the oculars, only the microphone.

OOSTERHUIS: In case my question is too tricky, do you think that others also can learn to operate the way you are doing without using the microscope?

BINKHORST: I certainly think anyone can as far as cataract surgery is concerned, and even the insertion of lenses and even if they have very fine loops or extensions, I do not think a microscope is needed. There are very good telescopic spectacles now, not only two times, but also three or four times, and I think that is more than enough for this type of surgery. But I agree that the young surgeons should train themselves with the microscope, because there are other types of surgery that need it badly. I think, keratoplasty, and other perhaps fine antiglaucoma operations. The disadvantage of using a microscope, I found that you lose the contact with the patient and also the contact with the eye and for me it is very important. Let me give an example: If a patient starts to move under an operation, it happens here and there, not in my hospital, you are not aware of it, something happens in the neighbourhood and you are not aware of it. But that is a very personal view and that is because I am too old to learn it.

OOSTERHUIS: May I ask the others of the panel of they all use the operating microscope, Dr. LEEMAN?

LEEMAN: I do not use them in cataract extractions. Of course I do in keratoplasty and glaucoma operations, but not in cataract extractions.

OOSTERHUIS: And Dr. JAFFE?

JAFFE: I am already being considered senile in my country because I had not changed to the microscope. I use loupes, $4\frac{1}{2}$ times with a wide angle, I have more than the width of the entire eyeball from canthus to canthus in these loupes. They are made by designs for vision. The big problem with the high magnification telescopic loupes is that your field is too small, but not with these. This is a large field, $4\frac{1}{2}$ times magnification. But to answer the original question: Should a young person and a young ophthalmologist start using the microscope? I think it would be really ludicrous to-day if he does not start using the microscope. There is no question that they will design devices, operations and useful operations that we never dreamed of. And the future in surgery will be microscopic surgery, this has been proven over and over again. However, the big criticism always is that somebody says: What are your results with the microscope compared to this one's results with the loupes, and you show no improvement. But that is not the point. The point is: When you see more and you see bigger and you learn to use the microscope better, you are more facile with it and you get better results and the young people should do this. The big problem is: What happens when a person at my age now, who has already done more than 10.000 cataract extractions over a period of 25 years, starts to use the microscope? There is no question that my patients will suffer for a certain period of time. If a man like Max FINE our foremost keratoplastic surgeon in the United States, can operate with loupes, and if a man like Dr. BINKHORST can operate with loupes, then why should I change to the microscope? I certainly feel more comfortable working with the loupes and use the microscope only for things like combined trabeculectomy cataract extractions and things of that nature. Otherwise I think we can do it well this way, but I still think that every young person should learn to use the microscope first before he does anything else.

OOSTERHUIS: Thank you. I am glad to hear that and I hope that everybody here who has in mind to start with implant surgery first starts to buy a microscope. I take this is also the opinion of Professor DRAEGER?

WORST: One technical point is that the lens must be inspected under the microscope before insertion to be sure that there are no foreign bodies attached to it. So in any case the microscope must be near the operative field.

DRAEGER: Just two little comments. You must not be afraid to lose the contact with a patient. If you have a very tiny little microscope, it takes a small place of your visual field, so you see your patient quite well at the side of your microscope, this is one point, so I would notice if the patient starts moving. We do not have the problem, as Dr. BINK-HORST also has not, as we do the serious cases under general anesthesia. But the other point, and this was not mentioned, is not only the magnification we talk about when we ask for a microscope, it is illumination too, and this is a very important point and you cannot combine a perfect illumination with a loupe. So this is another very important point which advocates the use of a microscope.

OOSTERHUIS: Thank you. Now we leave the microscope and I want to ask Jan WORST one question and this is the implant technique in glaucoma, when the patient has a glaucoma. We always hear about a very secure wound closure and will you tell me about it because I think this is a topic of your very special interest.

WORST: There are two situations, an existing bleb and the cataract where you want to preserve the bleb, in that case the extraction is done from below. It is an awkward technique, backbreaking and very difficult on the surgeon, but in that case it is quite possible to do the normal lens implantation technique and there is no difference it seems with what we call the normal lens implantation.

The second problem is the confirmed glaucoma which does not respond to topical miotics and Diamox. I do use a special suturing technique of my own, which is with steel sutures, and when the operation is finished between the middle two 12 o'clock sutures a Scheie operation is performed after which the conjunctival flap is sutured extremely carefully. And I feel that the loss of the anterior chamber is prevented by constructing so to say a second external anterior chamber below the conjunctival flap. I am not too much afraid in even combining the operation with a lens implantation. I do not remember having seen serious problems after this, but possibly a small hole falls in the conjunctiva, and I think the microscope will be very useful here to check up on every possible leak outside, because when there is a leak outside of the conjunctiva in the conjunctival sack it is the starting point for a flat anterior chamber. I have not very many cases but I find it a rather nice indication.

OOSTERHUIS: Thank you very much. Are there any others on the panel who have experience in this field? No? Well, thank you. I think I have one other question and one thing I do not understand. Norman JAFFE told us that the visual acuity which he obtained after implantation in a relatively younger group of people was lower than at the older age. Is that not true? Now, when I asked NORDLOHNE who made statistical studies how it is in material on BINK-HORST and WORST he told me that this is not the same in their series. I think this might be an important fact because I heard that perhaps the macular oedema which you can get after lens implantation as a complication might perhaps be related to the type of implant and I think at the moment we do not know, I just want to state that this lower visual acuity in your age group has not been observed in the two large series in Holland. Do you want to comment on that?

149

JAFFE: I can only accept that those are the facts if that is what
           they are, and nothing more. I still hold my original view
           that the implantation of the lens in a very presenile type
           of individual is an operation on an eye which is proto-
           plasmatically poor, is subject to more complications, the
           incidence of detachment of the retina is higher in these
           eyes, there must be reasons for these things, and therefore
           I consider that to be a hazardous eye. My series on these
           was obviously very small because of a gentlemen's agree-
           ment in the city of Miami not to do young people, but
           those that I managed to sneak in before the curtain was
           dropped showed me that these are cases that I should
           avoid. However, if it is shown by the series of BINK-
           HORST and the series of WORST that these eyes fare just
           as well I would say: fine, I would accept them if they
           are statistically verified facts and I have no reason to cri-
           ticise them. After all, if I have a relatively small series and
           their series is much larger than mine, then perhaps their
           facts are speaking louder than mine. But in any rate this
           has been my experience and I must say that I am very
           leery about operating on a young person. You know it
           really is a big problem. We have been talking about put-
           ting lenses in eyes and doing all these things and we really
           have not spoken about: does the patient really need a
           cataract extraction to begin with? And getting the idea
           that we are beginning to operate on all eyes that have
           cataracts? And this I must tell you: In the United States
           it has been a source, in all universities and all cities, a
           source of great contention, that some people seem to be
           doing too much cataract surgery, let alone implant surger-
           y. So we ought to try to make these decisions. The other
           thing that I would really like to ask is: What happened to
           the entity of phako-anaphylactic uveitis? Did it just dis-
           appear from the face of the earth? I just like to know.
           Does anybody see that in Holland or is this an entity that
           is seen only in other countries?

Voice: No, I do not think it exists as an entity.

JAFFE: Now that is of great interest to me, particularly when I
           have slides of lens material surrounded by three zones
           polymorpho-nuclear leucocytes surrounding lens material,
           a second circular zone of round cells, and a third zone of
           epitheloid and giant cells and degenerating plasma cells,
           the so-called Russell bodies, I presented pictures of these
           in my book, and these were not just from traumatic extra-
           capsulars, they were planned extracapsular extractions
           from our own pathological files. So I really wonder what
           has happened to the entity, should we just forget that we

ever learned it and tell the Irvines that when they classified it that that should be removed from the classification of lens induced inflammation, or what? But I know that we still see it in the United States.

OOSTERHUIS: Well, I think this is just like we discussed about the visual acuity in a different age group being different in the States as compared to our country. Now we proceed to the next question which I have to ask. One of the most serious problems is the corneal dystrophy and, well, there are quite a number of patients who have developed it and I want to know from you: How is the prognosis for the keratoplasty in these patients? I start with Jan. You have to wait for two years.

WORST: Now the situation has developed recently because of local changes in management of the hospital. Before, I must say that I am not a keratoplastic surgeon. I have to do them and I found some of the best results to occur in the implant cases. I consider it to have a quite good prognosis, but personally I would prefer to refer my cases to a centre where there is more experience with corneoplasty.

BINKHORST: I can only speak about the corneal dystrophies caused by endothelial contact and I have an idea about this, why the prognosis of keratoplasty in these cases is so good. I think it is because there is only a local damage of the endothelium, although the whole cornea may have become oedematous. And the cause of it is a local damage to the endothelium and if we do a keratoplasty we can eliminate that area of damaged endothelium and therefore I think the transplant has a better future than in a cornea with a generalized endothelial dystrophy.

OOSTERHUIS: Thank you. I am glad to say that in our clinic Dr. KOK-VAN ALPHEN performed keratoplasty in, I think, 9 cases and that in all cases the outcome was very favourable, so I agree completely with your comments and I hope that also Norman JAFFE can tell us that he has equally favourable results.

JAFFE: I will not use any more time. I agree completely. This is one of the most favourable types of cases for keratoplasty.

OOSTERHUIS: Thank you very much.

WORST: One technical point to the audience is that if this happens, the implant must not be removed.

JAFFE: Well, that is why it is good, because you leave the implant
                in place and the vitreous is kept back. I know with our
                type of implant it is impossible for the vitreous to turn
                the margin of the pupil to come into the anterior cham-
                ber, so it becomes one of the most favourable types of
                keratoplasty, and that has been my experience complete-
                ly.

OOSTERHUIS: Thank you very much. I think this is a very clear state-
                ment and this is very useful. I am very happy about it,
                because this is one of the serious complications and it
                means that these patients can be helped and can regain a
                useful, or even very good visual acuity. Now I want Dr.
                JAFFE to tell us about the cause of the macular disease
                he observed in such a large number of patients and what
                he thinks is the reason for it.

JAFFE: Well, in the first place I should preface this by saying that
                I do not know. And I will go beyond saying that I do not
                know by speculating, because now I am no longer talking
                about facts, I am giving what I criticised before, I am
                giving opinions now. So accept these merely as opinions
                and not facts. The problem of cystoid macular oedema
                has not been solved. From the time IRVINE described it
                in 1953 the only real advance that was made was made by
                J. DONALD GASS of our institution several years ago,
                when he was able to caracterize what the macular lesion
                looked like, caracterize the fluorescein pattern, and for
                caracterizing and suggesting the nature of the problem.
                For me cystoid macular oedema merely represents an end
                result of many, many different types of diseases, because
                cystoid macular oedema is not pathognomonic of the
                Irvine syndrome. It is seen, as you know, in diabetes
                mellitus, it is seen in central vein thrombosis, teleangiect-
                asia of the retina, it is seen in pars planitis, it is seen in
                aphakic patients with glaucoma occasionally who are
                treated with epinephrine, and now we are even learning
                that it is seen in a disease such as retinitis pigmentosa, and
                how could anybody imagine why it would occur in that?
                So there is a multiplicity of causes and a multivaried
                aetiology, but the end stage is cystoid macular oedema.
                Now in implant surgery the cystoid macular oedema we
                see is a response to intraocular inflammation and if you
                like to call this a vitreitis, if you will accept that termin-
                ology, that is what I would like to call it. There is no
                question when you examine these eyes you see an infil-
                tration of cells into the posterior detached vitreous and
                you sometimes see large, what we call V.P., just like the
                K.P., vitreous precipitates on the back of the detached

vitreous. So it is an inflammatory lesion. Now why whould we get an inflammatory lesion? I think the big problem is going to be settled. I know Jan has ideas about what causes this, I do not know yet, but at any rate, for me the reason cystoid macular oedema occurs more in cataract surgery and in implant surgery than in other types of intraocular surgery, such as glaucoma, retinal detachment surgery, keratoplasties in phakic eyes, is that we alter the structure of the vitreous. Jan was struggling a little bit with his anatomy before, if he gets out of the canal of Petit and gets into the space of Hannover, the space between the anterior and posterior zonular fibres which go circumferentially around the lens, that is one type of space. But I am concerned with the zonular fibres which rest on the intrahyloid membrane and go through the anterior part of the secondary vitreous and that encloses the what is really a potential space known as the canal of Petit, which I think you are familiar with. Now, at any rate I believe in cataract surgery that we lose the zonular support of the vitreous at the vitreous base and I believe that with the turbulence of the vitreous and the moving of the eye there is a greater pull on the vitreous base and it is this pull at the periphery of the retina and the pars plana, the shock, that causes cystoid macular oedema, because there seems to be a peculiar predilection for the association of diseases of the periphery of the retina and pars plana with cystoid macular oedema. So this is why I think patients get cystoid macular oedema. But I am sort of dodging the issue when I say: Why do you get it more with implant surgery than you do with other types of cases? I think theoretically the implant surgery should give you less cystoid macular oedema, because there is less vitreous shock. However, I think an additional factor is added, and I am just going to make it very simple for myself, I am saying that we have the aphakic eye with the disruption of some of the vitreous base, I am not saying it detaches but it becomes looser, plus the added factor of a foreign body inside that eyeball creating intraocular inflammation and perhaps an inpouring of cells into the eye, even though the eye looks white, and even though the eye looks relatively uninflamed. And I think that it is this added factor to the aphakic state that causes the cystoid macular oedema. I am now going to show my slides, Mr. chairman.

OOSTERHUIS: Thank you very much.

JAFFE: There you get the idea histologically in two slides representing cystoid macular oedema after cataract extrac-

153

tion. The lower slide is more typical because you certainly get the impression that these cystoid spaces intercommunicate and that little defect in the internal membrane is just in the preparation of the slide. The one above is also a case of cystoid macular oedema after cataract extraction, but from the histological point of view is not as typical as the one below. Next slide: I do not think this is showing too well. That certainly is the fluorescein pattern you are all familiar with, the pattern that you get showing the leakage of dye, and the leakage of dye comes, as you know, from the intraretinal capillaries.

Now we like to play a little game with our residents. We ask them to count the number of bubbles that they see, because the more you look, the more you see. Next slide: And this shows schematically the compartmentalization and we believe that this compartmentalization of the cystoid spaces is due to merely supporting fibres which probably connect the internal with the external membrane of the retina. Next slide. Now, it is going to be very difficult for you to see that, but this is a case of cystoid macular oedema photographed through the Hruby lens. Those of you who are up close enough to focus, and I cannot see it from here, there are little cystoid spaces which show this cystoid macular oedema. Next slide. And to show you why you must make this diagnosis first on a clinical basis without fluorescein, with a fundus contact lens or with a Hruby lens, is that this is what it normally looks like when you look with an ophthalmoscope, and this is with a direct ophthalmoscope. And you could see that there are two cystoid spaces connected with each other obliquely, but I assure you in this eye there was a multiplicity of little bubbles around these two larger ones that you saw. So you need this type of examination, it needed extra help to make the diagnosis. But I sustain what I said in the other cities that I spoke, you do not have to belong to a university, you do not have to have an elaborate photographic technique to make this diagnosis. If you are not sure what you are seeing in the macula, you can still give an intravenous injection of fluorescein and take the redfree filter of your indirect ophthalmoscope off and make the diagnosis.

WORST: Once a hypothesis starts explaining a large number of facts the moment comes that you are induced to form a theory. (Extended description of this theory is given in this book on page 159).

OOSTERHUIS: Thank you very much. Norman JAFFE can you tell us if this fits in well with your theory?

154

JAFFE: In the first place I believe, Jan, I see a number of facts that you presented and I see a number of opinions, and I must admit that it looks like the wildest scheme that I have ever seen in my life! However, let me answer. You know what Jan is talking about, you know it is like everything else, Jan is very ingenious and he had devised from his own observations a very great scheme and it is adventurous and I hope you will bear this in mind if you ever report this, that this exact work, as you know, was reported in the American Journal of Ophthalmology many years ago by C.C. Tain of the Manhattan Eye and Throat Hospital, who wrote on the destructive action of aqueous and in another paper on the destructive action of vitreous, that they both had proteolytic functions and toxicities. His work, however,, has not been reproduced in the United States in other laboratories and the work has fallen into disrepute, I will just tell you that, at major institutions.

Secondly, one fact that you gave was interesting, is that the macula is an unprotected area. The basement membrane over the macula is so attenuated it is almost non-existent, it is almost just like it is over the optic nerve. Tain carried this one step further, he really felt that glaucomatous excavation of the disc was due to this proteolytic action because the disc also was not covered by an internal limiting membrane. But Jan, I would like to ask you, what happens in a case of pupillary block when the aqueous becomes misdirected posteriorly and it gets into the retrovitreal space? Why in those cases don't we see cystoid macular oedema with any frequency and why don't you see it in a normal posterior vitreous detachment?

WORST: When you come to the essence of the theory I must warn you I have an answer for every attack.

JAFFE: I know that.

WORST: First of all, in normal posterior vitreous detachment the rest of the vitreous does not show that peculiar Gruyère cheese appearance, it has not formed sufficient holes and is the natural barrier between this area and the anterior chamber.

Second, your question about the acute glaucoma. It might very well be that it becomes acute because there is no posterior route and that all the aqueous remains dammed up in this big pocket in the front of the vitreous, while behind it there is no proper communication with the detached posterior vitreous. Nobody has seen this, nobody

155

knows it, it remains absolutely theoretical.

JAFFE: Jan that is not so. There is a misdirection of aqueous in pupillary block and it is aqueous with ABC in it.

WORST: When you see the drawings made by for instance BARRAQUER, you will see the pockets overhere and overhere, and you are supposed to do discission of these areas. You are not supposed to direct your needle, if I go by what the American Teaching says, you are not supposed to tap this, but you are supposed to tap this and this.

JAFFE: You are misinterpreting the American thinking, it is just the opposite. You create a communication between the anterior chamber and the retrovitreous space, and you must go through the posterior limiting border of the detached vitreous.

WORST: First of all this, O.K., one up for you!

OOSTERHUIS: Professor DRAEGER will be giving the final solution.

DRAEGER: Of course this is a very serious objection to your theory, Dr. WORST, one has to talk about especially in Holland. The cheese you refer to is Emmentaler.

OOSTERHUIS: I want to make only one remark about that and that is about the fluorescein angiography, because with fluorescein angiography this picture which you see, this leakage of the vessel is almost always related to some toxic reaction of the vessel wall, either to hypoxy and diabetes or little vein thrombosis, either to other toxic actions in pars planitis, and I think that anyhow it might from the fluorescein angiographic viewpoint very well be that a toxic action may be at least partly responsible for the development of this picture.

Now I think we come to the last topic that we will shortly discuss. We have first started, as you will know, with facts. We proceeded as you can see on the black board with suppositions, and we will end up with the unknown. And what is unknown is the future. The future of you sitting here. What will be the future of the implant lenses in Holland and in other countries? I think some short comments about that will be very worthwhile, perhaps after ten years when we read it again we will laugh at it, but anyhow I think at this moment it is very important. Now I heard that the residents in your institute and the residents in the clinic in Bremen, when they are very skilled are allowed to do implants, and I think in Holland, in Rotterdam as the only clinic in Holland this is also permitted. May I ask you what is your experience about that, what is your opinion about that. Do you think that this is, this can be part of the instruction of the residents? Professor DRAEGER.

DRAEGER: This is not a mandatory point of training. There are some senior residents which have a special skill in microsurgery who are allowed to do also implants, but this is not a fixed point in our training program. But we do not object having doing them some implants in their fourth year.

OOSTERHUIS: Yes, and Dr. JAFFE?

JAFFE: There is a semi-official policy now at the institute. We permit our senior residents, and there are 2 who go on to an extra year and it is those two who are permitted to do six implants each in their final year. We started that two years ago and it has been successful. Now this was a major change to the university. However, I must tell you that the residents in the United States generally, from what I hear speaking to many of the younger people, do a far greater number of cataract extractions during their residency program and training period, perhaps 6 or 7 times as many as are done here in the Netherlands. At least if the young people that I spoke to in the several days are representative, and I believe that they are. Just to put it in numbers: I believe that a resident at most institutions in the United States will do approximately 140 cataract extractions during his period and they will all be well instructed. I must tell you that under the most careful supervision and scrutiny Dr. DAVID CASSNER, the founder of vitrectomy, teaches the students at the beginning to do cataract surgery. He forces them to put in one suture only and make it a good one. He forces them to do ten sutures. He puts them through all types of little complications that they feel can be safely managed with the patient, so that they will be done under scrutiny. But you know JOHAN MACCLAINE, before he died, used to say, that the person who could do the best cataract extraction is his senior resident because he has done the most cataract surgery within the briefest period of time. I know in Holland you would all disagree with that, and I must say that I disagree with that too, but nevertheless it all depends on how well trained the resident is and how much surgery he has had. And since an institution like ours which was so anti-implant in 1966 to 1968 now permits the residents to do them this is an entire change in official

policy and I believe that a resident should leave our in-
stituation having performed intraocular lenses under careful supervision. That is my opinion.

OOSTERHUIS: Thank you very much. May I ask Dr. LEEMAN now
whether he has an opinion about this, especially as regards
the general ophthalmic surgeon here in Holland in his own
practice.

LEEMAN: Yes I have. To me it is a matter of great concern.
In my paper I already revealed the fact that in Holland we
have about 300 ophthalmologists of whom approxi-
matebly 200 do ophthalmic surgery. In our country there
are about 5000 cataractoperations to be done per year. So
every surgeon has an average of 25 cases. This may be just
enough to keep up ones surgical experience but in my
opinion it is not enough to do implant surgery. Therefore
I am of the opinion that implant surgery should be con-
centrated in a number of centers.

OOSTERHUIS: Thank you very much, I think this is a very clear state-
ment. And now, well, Dr. BINKHORST initiated this implant lenses and stimulated already 10% as he told, of the
Dutch ophthalmologists to follow the master and I think
the master has to tell us what is his opinion about it as
regards to the future.

BINKHORST: Partly I want to throw the ball back to you. As far as residents are concerned, I think it is the responsibility of the
university professors what they do and what they do not
do. But who is responsible for what the settled eye
surgeons do? Now of course everyone individually is responsible for his own work, but as a community of eye
surgeons I think the Dutch Ophthalmological Society
should feel responsible for what is happening in the
Netherlands in this respect especially and I cannot give
you the solution, I cannot answer your questions what
should be done, but may I suggest that a committee of the
Dutch Ophthalmological Society is installed to study this
problem? It is all I have to say.

OOSTERHUIS: Thank you. I think the most important is that we have to
decide what to do, that we have to think about it in the
future, and we have to find the best way.
Ladies and Gentlemen, this is the end of the panel discussion.

AQUEOUS HUMOUR BIOTOXICITY.

A unifying pathogenetic theory based on hypothetical aqueous
biotoxic factors.

J.G.F. WORST

(Haren, Gr.)

'C'est suivre l'example de ses maîtres de na pas toujours
les imiter'. (Hervouet)

INTRODUCTION

A number of physiological-, anatomical- and pathophysiological observations
gave us reason to assume that aqueous humour contains biochemically
active principles, which will manifest biotoxic effects when it leaves its
natural reservoir.
As a tentative name for these biotoxic principles the term Aqueous Biotoxic
Complex is proposed. (ABC factors).
A working hypothesis on the pathogenetic mechanism of ABC factors
tries to explain a number of apparantly unrelated pathological conditions by
bringing them under the common denominator of interstitial edema associated with capillary damage as caused by aqueous biotoxicity. ABC
factors do not manifest themselves under physiological conditions as the
walls of the aqueous reservoir offer active or passive protection.

THE AQUEOUS HUMOUR RESERVOIR.

The aqueous humour reservoir is formed by the anterior and posterior
chamber. Its anterior boundary is the corneal endothelium; the endothelium
has an active function in protecting the cornea from ABC factors. Inside
the aqueous humour reservoir the zonular fibers and the iris have an active
or passive inertness against ABC influences.
As the endothelial covering of the cornea is embryologically a mesothe-
lium and as also the iris is supposed to have a mesothelial covering, the
protective action of the surface layers of cornea and the anterior iris surface
might have the same biophysical basis. The pigment layer of the iris has a
protective function of its own against aqueous imbibition. The pigment, as
an ABC protecting layer, also plays a rôle in retinal detachment prevention.
The lens is particularly vulnerable to ABC influences but is effectively
separated from aqueous by the sub-capsular epithelium. The aqueous reservoir is filled with aqueous humour from the ciliary body and is emptied
through the trabecular meshwork (the filtration angle). Though the name

159

suggest a filtering function, little information exists on the nature of this filtration. In the context of the present ABC theory it is suggested that the corneo-scleral meshwork is concerned with [1]'de-toxicification' of aqueous humour. In this sense the trabecular meshwork functions as the kidney of the eye.

The posterior boundary of the aqueous humour reservoir is the anterior hyaloid membrane. Whether this is an actual membrane or merely a surface condensation of underlying vitreous body structures is irrelevant. From binocular microscope dissections and injections of corpusculate fluids and dyes in the posterior chamber one can conclude that the anterior vitreous surface is an impermeable membrane in the biophysical sense.

This membrane is often broken surgically during lens extraction. It does not regenerate its physical individuality. It had also been possible to remove the entire vitreous body behind the vitreous membrane leaving the membrane itself intact.

The vitreous membrane inserts on the posterior lens capsule as Wieger's hyaloideo-capsular ligament. This ligament is therefore the most distant recess of the aqueous humour reservoir.

Berger's retrolental space is not in direct communication with the posterior chamber aqueous reservoir.

INDICATIONS FOR THE PRESENCE OF ABC FACTORS IN AQUEOUS HUMOUR.

The most conspicious activity of aqueous humour is its degrading effects on the cornea when the protective endothelial layer becomes defective, by mechanical abrasion (lensimplantation with intermittent 'corneal touch syndrome') or by disease (Fuch's dystrophy or acute keratoconus).

Endothelial decompensation leads to aqueous imbibition, the formation of edema and finally irreversible disintegration of stromal substance (collagenolysis). Advanced dystrophies due to endothelial decompensation also show cystic changes in the epithelium.

A similar type of epithelial degeneration occurs in cases where a fistulizing procedure has resulted in external dripping of aqueous on the epithelium (luxuriant bleb after Elliot trephining). These stromal and epithelial degenerative phenomena form an indication that aqueous humour can exert biotoxic effects, and is far from being a 'simple' endocular 'lymph'.

AQUEOUS HUMOUR AND GLAUCOMA SURGERY.

Any succesful surgical intervention against glaucoma results in the formation of a 'fistula'. Anatomically this fistulous bleb consists of edematous spaces surrounded by severely degenerated connective tissue.

The capillary network around this bleb fails to invade the edematous cystic area and wound healing in the surgical area of a fistulizing area had been described as a collagenolytic activity. (TENG, CHI and KATZIN).

The failure of vascular ingrowth is interpreted here as due to an anti-vascular factor in the aqueous seeping into the cystic degenerative area. One of the possible ABC factors therefore could be a collagenolytic enzyme.

160

Another factor could be an anti-capillary agent or anti-endothelial agent which causes a disintegration of capillaries followed by local interstitial edema. In this context Prostaglandins might be a defendable guess.

The ABC effect on wound healing by inhibiting capillary growth and causing collagenolysis is also clinically evident in cataract wound healing when local wound dehiscence permits external aqueous flow. (The resulting anti-cicatricial powers of aqueous might also explain the inability of the iris to regenerate after surgical trauma, like an iridectomy or an iridotomy).

As further support of the presence of lytic enzymes in the anterior chamber one may quote the experiences with tissue transplantations on the iris for the purpose of intraocular tissue culturing. Any transplanted tissue in the anterior chamber will eventually become absorbed, whether freely floating in the aqueous humour or whether implanted on the iris surface.

BLOOD COAGULATING ABC FACTORS.

It is a well known surgical observation that blood entering the anterior chamber will rapidly coagulate. Aqueous obviously contains some form of coagulase. (Secondary aqueous lacks this capacity). The clinical fact of aqueous having blood coagulating properties raises a number of interesting physiological questions.

As aqueous leaves the anterior chamber by way of Schlemm's canal, which is a venous sinus, the admixture of aqueous humour with blood of the episcleral venous system (aqueous veins) should result in local thrombosis. As blood freely mixes with aqueous in the episcleral veins while it would coagulate in aqueous in the anterior chamber one must conclude that the composition of aqueous in Schlemm's canal differs from the composition of aqueous in the anterior chamber. In Schlemm's canal the coagulase of anterior chamber aqueous has been removed.

In the context of this hypothesis of ABC factors the filtration angle has performed a true filtering activity.

It is tempting to attribute this 'detoxifying' function to the highly specialized structures on the internal wall of Schlemm's canal. Aqueous humour might be 'processed' during the intra-cellular passage through SPEAKMAN's cells.

ABC FACTORS AND THE LENS.

Any small opening in the anterior capsule results in rapid swelling of lens fibers. This is the same effect as aqueous percolating through the corneal endothelium causes corneal swelling.

Aqueous imbibition results in a total destruction of all lens fibers and their final liquifaction and dissolution.

Secondary processes (anaphylaxia and inflammation) counteract the initial favourable lysis of lens matter by aqueous humour.

In principle however, the eye contains aqueous humour capable of removing lens fibers by enzymatic action. Therefore this must be one of the ABC factors. Whether this is the same factor which causes corneal edema or whether this a different one, is beyond the function of this hypothesis.

Teleologically speaking this anti-lens fiber enzyme is a highly useful component of the aqueous humour as in cases of lens trauma the eye contains its own curative agent.

It is in fact possible to make a good surgical use of this particular ABC effects on lens matter, by applying a discision, after which the lens fibers are attacked by the lytic action of aqueous, and can easily be washed out by irrigation, as a secondary procedure.

ABC FACTORS IN THE POSTERIOR SEGMENT.

Anatomically the aqueous humour reservoir is hermetically walled of from ABC factors by the anterior hyaloid membrane. From a number of physical experiments and anatomical dissections we have come to the conclusion that the anterior vitreous hyaloid is physically a highly impermeable membrane which in many respects resembles cellophane. It is the 'iron curtain' between the anterior and the posterior segment.

Embryologically speaking it is the boundary between the ectodermal and the entodermal part of the eye. It is the dividing line between the embryologicaL rallying point of neuro-dermal tissue (the retina) with skin tissue (the lens). (In developmental terms the lens has been called an ectodermal cyst (PLANTEN).

The posterior segment of the eye in this respect should be called an incomplete brain cyst. Also on embryological grounds it is possible that a strict physiological separation exists between these two structures. Metaphorically, the intracapsular extraction of the human lens is a neuro-surgical intervention for the eye, while the extracapsular removal of the lens is merely the opening of a dermoïd cyst.

Under normal physiological conditions the aqueous humour cannot enter the posterior segment. It is an essential supposition for this hypothesis that the physiological boundary of the anterior vitreous hyaloid surface is absolute for large molecular ABC factors. (It is permeable to f.i. fluorescein). If the toxic effects as proposed in this hypothesis are real, their entering the posterior segment would cause pathogenetic effects.

We have been able to observe a number of such effects in clinical cases, where it has been possible to compare right and left eyes with intact vitreous membranes on the one hand and broken anterior vitreous surfaces on the other hand. (Other clinical conditions being rigorously the same).

In the cases mentioned complete symmetry in anatomical aspect existed except for the disrupted hyaloid membrane. We have noticed: Unilateral vitritis; unilateral macular edema of the cystoid type (CMD) and last but not least: Retinal detachment.

Intracapsular lens extraction may cause disruption of the anterior surface of the hyaloid in an early or a late operative stage.

This disruption however is by no means symmetrical.

In lensimplantation cases in particular, it is a common occurrence that the vitreous surface of one eye remains intact while the vitreous surface of the other is mechanically disrupted. Based on such cases I have come to the conclusion that the mere presence of an anterior vitreous disruption whithout any other clinical difference from the other eye is sufficient to lead to complications in the posterior segment.

The most common sequence to this break in the anterior surface is cystoid macular edema, leading to Cystoid Macular Degeneration (CMD).

This observation differs essentially from the concept of traction strands being responsible for CMD. Such traction phenomena are rare and usually absent. The isolated appearance of holes in the anterior vitreous surface associated with cystoid macular edema, in the total absence of any inflammatory signs except the CMD itself is the pivotal observation on which the ABC theory of this paper rests.

Clinically all cases of CMD following intracapsular cataract surgery and with lens implantations show a destruction of the anterior vitreous surface. (However, not all cases of visible damage to the anterior vitreous surface show cystoid macular degeneration).

It must further be stressed that not all defects in the anterior hyaloid are visible. Only such defects as can be detected in a dilated pupil can be diagnosed. However, in the presence of an artificial lens most vitreous surface damage is in fact visible in the dilated pupil. simply because of the mechanical reason of the disruption, which is the damage done by the posterior loops of the lens. The function of the vitreous membrane and its failure to wall off ABC factors from entering the posterior segment is demonstrated in an 'experiment' unwillingly performed in lensimplantations. It has been noted that in our series of 1900 lens implantations the incidence of cystoid macular edema is higher than in a comparable series of non-implanted cases. While going over individual cases with cystoid macular edema we have noticed a constant occurrence of mechanically produced defects in the anterior hyaloid surface in cases of cystoid macular edema. Only cases with unilateral cystoid macular edema in bilaterally implanted cases have been taken to support this observation.

In the field of artificial lens implantation one large series exists in which an author unwillingly has produced a high incidence of cystoid macular edema by choosing a type of lens which is known to cause extensive damage to the anterior vitreous surface. We are referring to Epstein's 'Maltese Cross' lens, later called the Copeland Iris Plane lens. This lens has been noted to produce the formation of an artificial lens membrane, which seems to be a form of degeneration of the anterior vitreous surface. It also has been noted to produce breaks in the anterior vitreous surface at its extremities resting against the vitreous membrane. The formation of this typical artificial lens membrane in cases of 'Maltese Cross' lens implantation is completely absent in some 4000 cases of pupil supported lens implantations of the BINKHORST type. As in the series of the MIAMI group cystoid macular edema shows such a high percentage that the procedure has been abandoned for this reason, it is possible to conclude that unwillingly this 'experiment' has given strong support to the hypothesis that damage to the anterior vitreous surface is the main cause of cystoid macular edema. The accompanying iris damage may also have released an excess of ABC factors, f.i. Prostaglandins.

There exist other explanations of cystoid macular edema, in particular the presence of mechanical traction strands in the vitreous in case of vitreous loss or in case of incomplete posterior vitreous detachment, and finally 'inflammation'.

It is possible that these factors play a rôle, but it is much more likely that this pathological anatomical arrangement of the vitreous body is only a visible manifestation of a broken anterior vitreous surface. In particular strands running to the macula could be explained as traction phenomena but the histological demonstration of these strands is a grafical way of showing the absence of vitreous body around the traction area.

This absence of any visible struture is simply the histological demonstration of the presence of posterior vitreous detachment. It would be interesting to examine histological slides in the light of the above mentioned hypothesis. The most important point would be to examine the anatomical relations of the posterior detached area with defects in the anterior hyaloid membrane.

In the context of this hypothesis of aqueous causing retinal damage by ABC factors it is also of significance that cases of vitrectomy for various clinical and surgical reasons show a high incidence of macular degeneration.

Of great importance in this context is the observation by Binkhorst that in some 400 cases of extra capsular extraction (which leaves the 'iron curtain' between anterior and posterior segment completely intact), cystoid macular edema and retinal detachment have virtually disappeared. There is a great difference in the clinical sequence to intracapsular versus extracapsular in relation to cystoid macular edema. This difference is so obvious that a 'statistical' survey is hardly necessary. (In this respect the phako-emulsification cannot be called a strictly extracapsular procedure).

As a further support for this membrane function of the posterior lens capsule, including the anterior vitreous hyaloid, one may quote the case of 'succesful' discission of an opaque posterior capsule, which result in a clear central hole, but is later followed by cystoid macular edema. Also in cases of phako-emulsification it is the author's assumption that breaking of the posterior capsule or the zonule will put the case in the category of the potential cystoid macular edema category. The suction device of the phako-emulsifier further is a potential risk for peripheral posterior capsule ruptures and zonular breaks. If the hypothesis that aqueous in Schlemm's canal differs from aqueous in the anterior chamber is correct it will be necessary to perform a micro-chemical analysis of aqueous humour in the anterior chamber and of aqueous humour emerging from the aqueous veins.

ANTI-COAGULATING OR HEMOLYTIC FACTORS IN THE AQUEOUS

Anterior chamber hemorrhages, post-operative or traumatic, are' dissolved by hemolysis, and blood clots in the anterior chamber will disappear. Aqueous therefore must contain hemolytic and anti-coagulant factors. Such agents would fall in the category of ABC factors. In view of the importance attributed to the anterior vitreous surface the following clinical observation could be of some significance: while blood in the anterior chamber is rapidly absorbed, the same blood, if trapped in the vitreous (even when prolapsed in the anterior chamber) but separated from the aqueous by an intact vitreous surface will take several weeks to be absorbed. Evidently the anterior hyaloid membrane is an effective partitioning between the blood dissolving factors of the aqueous and the blood behind the membrane.

One type of hemorrhage occurs, which does not coagulate in aqueous. It is the hemorrhage from Schlemm's canal as it occurs during rapid decompression. This unclottable hemorrhage is a clinical indication that the blood in Schlemm's canal has a different composition from blood which enters the anterior chamber by a surgical route.

Of the ABC factors the clotting factor must have been removed by the trabecular meshwork. Anti-coagulant factors however must have been added otherwise the reflux of Schlemm's canal blood should show coagulation, when re-entering the anterior chamber.

The simultaneous precence of clotting factors and anti-coagulants in the aqueous humour of the anterior chamber in Schlemm's canal is an intriguing problem which deserves further analysis. It is assumed that the anatomical and sub-microscopical configuration of the trabecular meshwork suggests an active bio-physical and bio-chemical rôle in 'processing' the aqueous humour.

In summary we have, from a number of general clinical observations, derived the presence of the following hypothetical ABCfactors;

1. A collagenolytic enzyme (Collagenolysine).
2. Blood coagulating substances (Coagulases).
3. Anti-coagulating substances (Hemolysins).
4. Anti-capillary substances.
5. Edema producing factors.

It would be tempting to ascribe the latter two effects to Prostaglandins. If Prostaglandins are present in the aqueous humour in physiological or in particular cases in pathological quantities (see: Iris Plane Lens and macular degeneration, page 163) it would be possible to explain cystoid macular degeneration (CMD) on the basis of the presence of Prostaglandins in the posterior vitreous detachment reservoir.

It may be of particular significance in this respect that the anti-prostaglandinase activity of Indomethacin has been used, on the basis of the above hypothetical Prostaglandin effect in CMD, by TENNANT, who has found a curative effect. IRVINE also has noticed a favourable effect of Indomethacin (Indocid) on Cystoid Macular Edema (CME).

The following clinical observations supports the thesis that the partition between the anterior and posterior chamber must be maintained in order to prevent CMD. Extracapsular lens extractions show a very low incidence of CMD. (BINKHORST). Aphakia through intracapsular surgery however, is a most effective way to open up the posterior segment to ABC factors, unless the anterior vitreous membrane remains intact. Intracapsular aphakia and CMD are related. Structures which are anatomically completely out of reach of ABC factors may under specific circumstances be exposed to them. Even the chorioid can be exposed to aqueous humour in case defects are present in the retina and the retinal pigment layer. (see: ABC factors and retinal detachment).

THE VITREOUS AND ABC DEGENERATIVE
EFFECTS

It is a not unfrequent observation in lensimplantation that a vitreous prolaps in the anterior chamber, be it around the artificial lens or moving freely through the iridectomy becomes progressively cloudy in a typical fashion. Also vitreous body inside the pupil and in particular the vitreous body in the periphery behind the iris root may, after cataract extraction with or without lensimplantation , show a typical 'murkiness'. It can be interpreted as a form of precipitation of the vitreous gel. It would be easy to interpret this vitreous opacification as a form of 'vitritis' suggesting an inflammatory factor. Most of these cases however show this phenomenon without convincing signs of inflammation. Clinically these cases with murky vitreous are potential cystoid macular edema cases, and some of them will end up with a retinal aphakic detachment.

The typical degeneration of the vitreous body is attributed by us hypothetically to ABC effects, in the sense that normal components of the aqueous humour are responsible for a destructive action on the vitreous body and retinal structures. The question may be raised why not all vitreous is subject to aqueous degeneration effects after cataract extraction. In case of an intact vitreous membrane no such effect can occur. In case of a broken vitreous membrane it seems that vitreous bodies which already show degeneration are more vulnerable to aqueous imbibition, while an intact hyaloid gel may ward of ABC influences.

In aphakia the base of the vitreous body and the peripheral retina are particularly exposed to ABC effects because of mechanical damage following intracapsular lensextraction. In anatomical specimens obtained several years after cataract extraction we noticed permanent damage because of intracapsular surgery. In particular breaks in the anterior vitreous surface are present as well as small retinal breaks at the ora-serrata, including the pigment layer.

Cystic changes resembling CMD in the retinal periphery are also frequent. It is postulated here that the entry of aqueous humour through the peripheral breaks in the anterior vitreous surface and through the pigment layer defect of the retinal periphery and the accompanying retinal breaks at the ora-serrata will lead to capillary damage of the chorio- capillaris. This ABC effect on the peripheral chorioid results in edema. In this context it is the anti-capillary factor or edema producing factor (Prostaglandins?) which cause aphakic detachment, by producing epichorioidal (= subretinal) fluid production.

The chorioidal capillaries are by their very nature highly vulnerable to contact with the anti-vascular ABC factors (Prostaglandins?). The same mechanism is supposed to play an essential rôle in the production of subretinal fluid in idiopathic retinal detachment, in the presence of a retinal tear. The hypothetical effect of aqueous on aphakic detachment refers to cases with extremely periferal retinal breaks which usually are difficult or impossible to be diagnosed by indirect ophthalmoscopy, even with indentation.

166

In a typical case of idiopathic retinal detachment the anatomical situation is the following: There is vitreous degeneration with liquefaction and cavity formation in the vitreous gel. The posterior vitreous is contracted leaving a free space (posterior vitreous detachment).

The posterior vitreous membrane is intact except over the area detached from the optic nerve, which forms a real hole. Cloquet's canal communicates with the posterior vitreous detachment reservoir, by way of the posterior vitreous 'ring'. It is highly probable that the fluid reservoir of the posterior vitreous detachment communicates freely with the anterior vitreous body and with the aqueous in the posterior chamber. This configuration was observed in injection experiments by the author, using particulate matter and using injections of white India ink in the posterior chamber of senile eyes with posterior vitreous detachment. Some ink particles will find their way through breaks in the peripheral anterior vitreous surface and reach the posterior vitreous detachment reservoir by way of a circuitous route through the degenerated vitreous body. This type of vitreous body may be compared to Gruyère cheese. (PROF. DRAEGER had kindly redefined this as Emmenthaler cheese...). It is assumed that the progressive 'cavitation' of aphakic vitreous is an ABC determined degenerative phenomenon.

The presence of aqueous humour in the posterior vitreous detachment reservoir is generally inocuous. In conditions where the anterior limiting membrane of the retina is defective however, vascular damage of the type as induced by the ABC factors can occur.

There are at least three points in the retina where such ABC effect on vascular structures can manifest itself:

1. On the optic nerve head.
2. In the macular area.
3. Through defects in the retinal surface, in the form of retinal degenerations or manifest retinal tears.

1. In case of contact of the optic nerve head with ABC factors some local edema may be expected.
2. In case of contact of the macula with ABC factors cystoid macular edema will set in. It must be noted that in fluoresceine studies of cystoid macular edema the presence of optic nerve head edema is not infrequent. An explanation of this association is usually omitted.
3. A possible explanation of the high vulnerability of the macula to ABC factors could be the anatomical configuration of the internal limiting membrane. This internal limiting membrane at the foveal periphery measures 1500 Mμ. However, the exact center of the macula has an internal limiting membrane thickness of 10-20 Mμ only. This signifies a reduction of thickness of a probably very important separating membrane of 1500 to ± 15 Mμ (JAFFE). In this sense the macula is a bare spot in the retina.
4. Retinal defects and aqueous ABC effects on the chorioid. An even barer spot in the retina is the manifest retinal hole, with or without retinal detachment, in case the retinal hole communicates directly with the ABC filled

posterior vitreous detachment reservoir or indirectly by way of the circuitous routes of the 'Gruyère cheese' cavitated vitreous body ABC factors will cause the capillary network of chorioidal capillaries to react in the standard manner with formation of edema. The edema producing effects of ABC factors herewith is considered the same whether exerted on the chorioidal capillaries or the capillaries of the macula or the optic nerve head.

In the light of the ABC hypothesis retinal detachment is a process of subretinal (epi-chorioidal) fluid formation caused by aqueous contact with the choriocapillaris through the retina and the pigment layer. The scleral sectional atrophy underlying retinal holes might be the deepest manifestation of ABC effects through the retinal defect. The above theory offers a good explanation of the absence of retinal detachment in many cases of manifest retinal holes. In this patho-genetic theory of retinal detachment the hole is only an essential link in a chain of events. Only when the hole serves as a point of entry for aqueous humour to the chorioid, retinal detachment will set in. If the overlying vitreous body is anatomically intact without cavitations, aqueous cannot reach the chorioid and retinal detachment cannot occur.

It is the anatomical configuration of the vitreous body and the posterior vitreous detachment in relation to the anatomical position of the hole, which determines whether this hole will be a potential retinal detachment hole or simply a defect in the retina without clinical significance in terms of later retinal detachment.

The hypothesis as proposed here is that the anatomical condition of the vitreous body in terms of permeability for aqueous ABC factors towards the retinal defects is the essential pathogenetic constellation of retinal detachment. This also offers an explanation for the therapeutic effects of certain retinal detachment operations: It has been noted that it is sufficient to produce a buckle under the chorioid without drainage of subretinal fluid to obtain a re-attachment of the retina in 24-28 hours. In terms of the hypothesis just exposed this could be interpreted as follows: The buckle walls off such intra-vitreal channels as gave access of aqueous to the choroid, closing off the vitreous holes, and preventing ABC factors from causing chorioidal edema. The additional treatment of the buckle area with either diathermy or freezing results in atrophy of the chorio-capillaris, wherewith the production of epi-chorioidal fluid (sub-retinal fluid) is stopped. The effect of a cerclage operation on aphakic detachments and other conditions could be explained by the constriction of the vitreous body in the equator, which leads to a constriction of all trans-vitreal exit channels of the aqueous humour.

Hypothetical though this ABC effect on retinal detachment may seem it must be born in mind that in any case of retinal detachment the intraocular pressure drops suddenly at the onset of retinal detachment. This drop in intraocular pressure with the onset of retinal detachment may simply signify that a second outflow passage has been opened.

The choriocapillaris in this respect functions in the same manner as the capillary bed around an edematous fistula. After successful retinal detachment surgery, even when simple diathermy has been applied over the area underlying the retinal defect the intraocular pressure will rise again to normal levels. This can be explained by assuming that the chorio-capillaris has been destroyed and entry of aqueous has been abolished by scar formation under the retinal hole. The occlusion of the retinal hole in the scar is a second highly effective way to wall of ABC factors.

SUMMARY

A hypothesis is proposed attributing a number of biotoxic effects to aqueous humour. (ABC — Aqueous Biotoxic Complex). Under normal anatomical and physiological conditions aqueous humour is contained in the anterior and posterior chamber reservoir and the ABC effects remain silent because the boundaries of the aqueous humour reservoir are resistant to these biotoxic factors. These factors are biochemically undefined but fall in the category of collagenolysins and anti-vascular enzymes. (Prostaglandins?) Outside the normal reservoir these biotoxic effects result in a specific pathology, like corneal edema, subconjunctival edema, lens fiber edema, macular edema, papilledema and chorioidal edema. (= retinal detachment).

Author's address:
J.G.F. WORST, M.D.
Department of Ophthalmology
Refaja Hospital
Stadskanaal
The Netherlands
Home address:
Julianalaan 11
Haren (Gr.)
The Netherlands